PRAISE FOR ANN LOUISE GITTLEMAN

"I deeply respect and honor the work of Ann Louise Gittleman, whom I consider as a teacher, as well as what she has done to bring intelligence to the world of nutrition."

—**Dr. Mark Hyman**, Medical Director of Cleveland Clinic's Center for Functional Medicine, and #1 *New York Times* bestselling author, including his latest book, *Food: WTF Should I Eat?*

"Ann Louise Gittleman is a dynamic pioneer and leading authority in nutrition, health, and wellness. She is a beacon of light and inspiration for millions of people who seek advanced healing information that genuinely transforms their lives."

—**Anthony William**, #1 *New York Times* bestselling author of *Medical Medium Liver Rescue: Answers to Eczema, Psoriasis, Diabetes, Strep, Acne, Gout, Bloating, Gallstones, Adrenal Stress, Fatigue, Fatty Liver, Weight Issues, SIBO & Autoimmune Disease*

"Rather than accepting conventional wisdom, Ann Louise is always light years ahead of it. Every time I read her books or attend her talks, I discover something new—whether it's state-of-the-art strategies for dealing with menopause, powerful detox techniques, or the hidden effects of parasites on our health. She never stops researching, never stops learning, and never stops advancing our field. I am continually awed by the depth and scope of her knowledge."

—**Dr. Kellyann Petrucci**, *New York Times* bestselling author of *10-Day Belly Slimdown*, and creator of drkellyann.com

"From Fat Flush to detox, Ann Louise Gittleman is a trailblazer whose impeccable, groundbreaking research and knowledge paved the path for nutritionists today. As she has for the past few decades, Gittleman continues to inspire, motivate, and challenge me today."

—**J. J. Virgin**, celebrity nutrition and fitness expert and *New York Times* bestselling author of *Warrior Mom: 7 Secrets to Bold, Brave Resilience*

"Ann Louise Gittleman, PhD, CNS, is a visionary and pioneer in the world of natural healing. Her bestselling books have revolutionized natural medicine and Ann Louise continues to innovate."

—**Izabella Wentz**, PharmD, FASCP-Functional Pharmacist and #1 *New York Times* bestselling author of *Hashimoto's Protocol* and *Hashimoto's the Root Cause*

"Ann Louise Gittleman has been a leading innovator in the field of integrative medicine for decades. Her books bring cutting-edge research to health consumers in an easy-to-understand form. She was one of the first to warn of the dangers of our infatuation with low-carb diets, and now science has validated her message."

—**Dr. Ronald Hoffman**, host of "Intelligent Medicine"

"Ann Louise Gittleman has done us all a service by showing how the essential fats can and should be used in an overall program for living longer, losing weight, and reaching optimal health."

—**Dr. Julian Whitaker**, Whitaker Wellness Institute

"Ann Louise Gittleman is to be commended for getting the detox message out to mainstream Americans. I couldn't agree more with her message and her methods."

—**Dr. Elson M. Haas**, author of *Staying Healthy with New Medicine*

"I have been privileged to know Ann Louise Gittleman for a number of decades and respect her dedication to assisting others achieve vibrant health with nutrition and natural therapies. She is truly at the top of her field, deserving designation as 'The First Lady of Nutrition'."

—**Dr. Jonathan V. Wright**, Medical Director, Tahoma Clinic, Tukwila, Washington

"Ann Louise Gittleman is the real deal. With her wealth of clinical experience and encyclopedic knowledge of nutrition and health she has been one of the great influences on my professional life and one of the first people I turn to when I want a 'second opinion'."

—**Jonny Bowden**, PhD, CNS, author of *The 150 Healthiest Foods on Earth*

"Ann Louise Gittleman has demonstrated extraordinary leadership when it comes to reporting on the fundamental causes of illness and disease. Whether it's parasites in *Guess What Came to Dinner?* or environmental toxins in *The Fat Flush Plan* or toxic EMF or RF in *Zapped*, she reaches the hearts of the public by not only demonstrating what causes illness but she also offers solutions on how to fix them! I'm proud to be one of her colleagues."

—**Dr. Stephen Sinatra**, integrative cardiologist and author of *The Sinatra Solution: Metabolic Cardiology*

"I recall interviewing her on the radio when I was just starting out in the field of nutritional medicine. . . . I was terrified because she was so much more knowledgeable than I. . . . So I read all her books and became even more impressed. She was one of the greats even back then. She continues to learn, explore, and, best of all, get the message out to millions of adoring fans."

—**Dr. Fred Pescatore**, author of *The A-List Diet: Lose up to 15 Pounds and Look and Feel Younger in Just 2 Weeks*

"A powerful 'Force of Nature' in the healing community, Ann Louise is used to being on the cutting edge. Want to see what the experts will be saying in twenty-five years? Simply see what she is saying NOW!"

—**Dr. Jacob Teitelbaum**, author of *The Fatigue and Fibromyalgia Solution*

"A long-time guiding light in the world of nutritional medicine, Ann Louise continues to be The First Lady of Nutrition and someone I can always count on for the best information for my patients, my readers, and me. Not only is she knowledgeable and a pioneer in the field, but she is a truly caring person who is dedicated to changing the world, one body at a time. I'm proud to call her my friend."

—**Dr. Hyla Cass**, author of *8 Weeks to Vibrant Health*

"I always admired her passion for healing for all, her desire to look deeper, and her healing wisdom."

—**Dr. Raphael Kellman**, of the Kellman Center for Functional and Integrative Medicine and author of *The Whole Brain: The Microbiome Solution to Heal Depression, Anxiety, and Mental Fog without Prescription Drugs*

"Ann Louise has always been one of my favorite go-to nutritionists. Her *Fat Flush Plan* and other programs, supplements, and test kits have paved the way for a whole new generation of health and environmentally like-minded advocates and activists. She is STILL a superstar in our changing world and we are all very grateful for her tireless efforts to bring the most cutting-edge wisdom to a world that desperately needs it."

—**Donna Gates**, Med, ABAAHP, Advanced Fellow with the American Academy of Anti-Aging Medicine and author of several books, including the international bestseller *The Body Ecology Diet: Recovering Your Health and Rebuilding Your Immunity*

"Ann Louise is ahead of the nutrition curve. She's always been cutting-edge in her approach, having been part of the lineage of nutritional mentors and pioneers who ultimately led the charge forward to the rise in the current twenty-first century health and wellness interests. I am grateful for her courage, for speaking the truth, and being holistically minded in all she writes, speaks, and champions in her work."

—**Deanna Minich**, PhD, FACN, CNS, IFMCP, nutritionist and author of *The Rainbow Diet*

"When it comes to wellness through nutrition, Ann Louise Gittleman not only pioneered the field, she continues to be ahead of her time and on top of the game. At *First for Women*, we rely on Gittleman to alert us to the newest scientific studies with the most urgent relevance for our readers—and she always delivers."

—**Carol Brooks**, editor in chief of *First for Women* and *Simple Grace* magazines

"Ann Louise's *Fat Flush Plan* is dietary common sense for all the right reasons—it's balanced, it's a program you can safely stay on for life, and it works."

—**Dr. Barry Sears**, *New York Times* bestselling author of *The Zone*

"Over the years, Ann Louise has always been at the forefront when it comes to nutrition for optimal health and weight loss. As a guest on my radio show, she frequently and generously shared her knowledge and cutting-edge advice with my listeners, answering their questions and discussing all aspects of healthy eating for both general health and healthy weight loss. I incorporated her *Fat Flush Plan* into my popular Fit Camps with successful results and was honored to coauthor *The Fat Flush Fitness Plan*. In a world where advice can be so questionable, Ann Louise continues to offer sound advice."

—**Joanie Greggains**, radio host and health and fitness educator

"Ann Louise Gittleman is an accomplished nutritionist, natural health educator and author with more insight into today's most prevalent health conditions than the typical MD. We need to be encouraging the leading voices in health, like Ann Louise Gittleman, who are the Paul Reveres of this generation. . . . "

—**Camilla Rees**, CEO of Wide Angle Health, LLC

"Ann Louise is one of the most intelligent, state-of-the-art nutritionists who is always sharing top-notch and innovative research in her books, with her supplements, and in everything she does. She is driven to share with the world the truth behind nutrition. Her programs and her books withstand the test of time and she will continue to be a leader in the industry. She is a rare gem and we should consider ourselves blessed to have her commitment to cutting-edge strategies for health and wellness."

—**Rachel Feldman**, owner of rachelafeldman.com, health coach and business coach, contributor at *Forbes*, *Huffington Post* and *Thrive Journal*

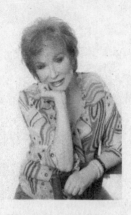

Photograph by Mark Huender

Ann Louise Gittleman holds an MS in Nutrition Education from Columbia University, US, the title of Certified Nutrition Specialist (CNS) from the American College of Nutrition, and a PhD in Holistic Nutrition. The bestselling author of more than thirty books, Gittleman has also served as the Chief Nutritionist of the Pediatric Clinic at Bellevue Hospital and is the former Director of Nutrition at the Pritikin Longevity Center in Santa Monica, California. She currently sits on the Advisory Board for the International Institute for Building-Biology & Ecology, the Nutritional Therapy Association, Inc., and Clear Passage, Inc.

For more information, please visit AnnLouise.com.

ALSO BY
ANN LOUISE GITTLEMAN, PHD, CNS

RADICAL
METABOLISM

A POWERFUL PLAN TO BLAST FAT
AND REIGNITE YOUR ENERGY
IN JUST 21 DAYS

BY ANN LOUISE GITTLEMAN, PHD, CNS
WITH VALERIE J. BURKE, MSN

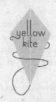

yellow
kite

First published in the United States of America by Da Capo Press, an imprint of Perseus Books, LLC, a subsidiary of Hachette Book Group, Inc.

First published in Great Britain in 2018 by Yellow Kite
An imprint of Hodder & Stoughton
An Hachette UK company

This paperback edition published in 2019

1

A CIP catalogue record for this title is available from the British Library

Paperback ISBN 978 1 529 37093 5

Printed and bound in Great Britain by Clays Ltd, Elcograf S.p.A

Hodder & Stoughton policy is to use papers that are natural, renewable and recyclable products and made from wood grown in sustainable forests. The logging and manufacturing processes are expected to conform to the environmental regulations of the country of origin.

Hodder & Stoughton Ltd
Carmelite House
50 Victoria Embankment
London EC4Y 0DZ

www.yellowkitebooks.co.uk

This book is lovingly dedicated to
Edith and Arthur Gittleman,
my cheerleaders in heaven.

CONTENTS

WHY I WROTE THIS BOOK

> Be fearless in the pursuit of what sets your soul on fire.
>
> —Unknown

Pembroke Branch Tel. 6689575

Please do me a favor.

I want you to throw out everything you thought you knew about health and weight loss. What you're about to read in this book will undoubtedly fly in the face of both conventional and even alternative dietary wisdom. But regardless of what you've tried before, get ready for a radical shift in your health. Because what we are doing is clearly not working—*we need a different plan, and we need it now.*

Westernized societies continue to grow fatter, sicker, and more toxic, but it isn't for lack of effort. About 60 percent of Americans are desperately trying to lose weight, yet only 5 to 10 percent actually keep it off. In 2013, the US spent $60.5 billion on weight-loss products and services alone.[1] You would think that with this many people investing that much money in their health, Americans would be the leanest and healthiest country on Earth, but nothing could be further from the truth. *Instead, we are world leaders in obesity and chronic disease.*

More than a third of us are obese, and the incidence of type 2 diabetes is going through the roof, with Alzheimer's disease not far behind. For the first time in decades, in 2015 US life expectancy *dropped* due to increased deaths from heart disease, stroke, Alzheimer's, diabetes, and kidney disease. In the United States, one in two women and one in three men will develop cancer in their lifetime. Not to mention the many common symptoms that so many of us live with every day, such as fatigue, indigestion, and depression.

Many clients come to me after having dieted for decades. In fact, even though nutritional advice has come a long way since the 1980s, these days many of you are struggling in spite of doing everything "right." Your weight-loss efforts have failed miserably despite eating clean, going gluten-free, and loading up on bone broth. This book reveals why and provides the necessary course correction.

Maybe you've even tried some of the latest diets, such as Keto, where the focus is on eating the way our ancestors presumably did. There is much to be said in praise of the direction these diets have taken us—specifically, moving refined sugar, gluten, and excess carbs aside in favor of more protein and fat. But there are pitfalls. Today our bodies have a hard time digesting fats, which causes digestive symptoms. People experience difficulty sustaining energy levels and losing excess weight. *Radical Metabolism* connects the dots for you in a powerful new way. You can think of it as the next wave—going beyond Keto, Paleo, and primal-style diets.

The current health statistics are staggering, but there *is* hope! You don't have to be a statistic. My intention is to bring you newly discovered secrets for reigniting a stalled metabolism, harmonizing your hormones, and healing your gut. It's no secret that obesity and chronic illness go hand in hand. Not only will I lay out a plan to re-energize your sluggish metabolism, but I will also provide some long overdue insights into all those mystery illnesses that are lumped together under "autoimmune conditions," which afflict millions of people today. I want this book to rock your world and reset your personal healing trajectory so that it's the last weight-loss book you'll ever need.

REWRITING THE RULES OF NUTRITION

Who am I, and why should you listen to me? For well over thirty years, I've been challenging conventional medicine and sharing the latest cutting-edge remedies. In 1988, I was reluctantly thrust onto the national stage with the publication of my first book. Later, as an award-winning *New York Times* bestselling author, my integrative and functional medicine colleagues called me a "visionary health expert" and "health pioneer." Over the course of my career, I have been deeply honored to be cited as one of the "Ten Most Knowledgeable Nutritionists" in the United States by *Self* magazine, received the Excellence in Medical Communication Award from the American Medical Writers Association, and was presented in 2016 with the Humanitarian Award by the Cancer Control Society.

I am an outside-of-the-box nutritionist! Back in the 1980s, everyone was munching on carbs and only carbs—Shredded Wheat and Grape-Nuts, to be exact—while eschewing any morsel of fat. I openly defied the reigning high-grain, high-carb, low-fat dietary recommendations of the time with my first book, *Beyond Pritikin* (the no- to low-fat Pritikin diet was the big health regimen back then). In my book, I proposed a new diet model featuring essential *fats* for weight loss, heart health, and immunity. This was downright health heresy at the time, but today the importance of healthy fats is widely acknowledged. After my departure from the Pritikin principles, noted health guru Dr. Robert Atkins invited me to appear as a regular on his radio shows on WOR in New York City, eventually asking me to run the diet department of his integrative medicine clinic in New York.

Shortly thereafter, I wrote *Super Nutrition for Women*, which further chastised carbohydrates and promoted a high-fat diet, this time for hormone health. I was the first to discuss nutritional strategies for perimenopause in my *New York Times* bestseller *Before the Change*. As early as 1997, I warned about the dangers of gluten in *Your Body Knows Best* and sounded the alarm about environmental toxicity, long before the terms *gluten-free* and *detox* were part of the American lexicon.

In 2002, I published the book for which I'm probably best known, *The Fat Flush Plan*. In *Fat Flush*, I introduced the importance of cleansing and focused on the liver as a primary fat-burning organ and detoxifier—diet heresy, once again, according to the *New York Times*. Yet, the book struck a long and enduring chord with the public and spawned a family of five additional titles. Since that time, hundreds of books about liver toxicity and detox and cleansing have appeared on bookstore shelves. In 2016, I even released a new updated version, *The New Fat Flush Plan*.

I've tirelessly searched to uncover root causes and hidden factors that sabotage weight loss and health. In *Guess What Came to Dinner?*, I also wrote about how parasites are not just a third-world problem: how they're masquerading as more commonly recognized conditions, such as weight-loss resistance, metabolic syndrome, bloating, inflammation, and chronic fatigue. I wrote about natural alternatives for menopause at a time when physicians were medicating women as if menopause itself were a disease. After publishing *The Fast Track Detox Diet* in 2005, I was featured on *20/20* for daring to say that chemicals, such as BPA, were making us fat. Of course today, the toxic effects of xenoestrogens and obesogens are widely accepted by mainstream medicine. In 2010, I took on the often overlooked and controversial biological risks of electropollution from Wi-Fi, mobile phones, and smart meters in my book *Zapped* and alluded to how connection addiction may be rewiring our brains and invisibly undermining our bodies.

For the last three decades I have found myself rewriting the rules of nutrition—and now, with *Radical Metabolism*, I'm at it again. Why? Because the latest science paints a new picture, and it's not a pretty one. I am well past fifty, and in moving through that transition I was personally challenged by a metabolic slowdown. The plan in this book has evolved from my discovery of what worked for me and others. I happily report that your metabolism can be reignited regardless of your age and exposure to environmental pollutants.

We are living a new toxic nightmare and the old remedies don't work. Every day we face an invisible war deep within our bodies as hormone-disrupting environmental pollutants contaminate, and progressively erode, our cellular defenses. Petrochemicals, plastics, heavy metals, fake hormones, radiation, microbes, and other toxic agents all wreak hormone havoc on our biology. Most of these toxins are hidden, lurking in our food, air, and water, as well as body care, household, and cleaning products, and even technology, which makes them even more insidious. This is not your parents' or grandparents' world anymore. Our planet—and our bodies—are crying out for help.

We have more than 37 trillion cells in the body, and every one of them is at risk. Once enough of your cells become compromised, then your tissue and organ function will soon follow. Healthy cells begin with healthy cell membranes. Without them, your body essentially stands naked and defenseless against those toxic assaults, which results in hormone disruption and inflammation. Inflammation is the number-one factor driving nearly every chronic disease today.

Back in 1858, physician Rudolf Virchow, the "father of modern pathology," said, "All diseases are disturbances at the cellular level." He argued that to treat a disease, we must first understand the cause—*and the cause is always found at the level of the cell.* There are many examples. Alzheimer's disease involves defective processing of amyloid precursor proteins by cells in the brain. A genetic predisposition to high cholesterol is caused by defective cellular uptake of lipoproteins. Cancer occurs when cells develop aberrant growth patterns, and autoimmune diseases arise when cellular communication runs amok.

And so it is with metabolism.

After working with literally thousands of "fat, forty, and fatigued" females, the pieces of the puzzle began to fall into place for me. It became clear that no diet in the world will work if your metabolism has turned toxic. One reason many diets fail is they don't correct the shutdown of key fat-burning tissues in the body. You have three important metabolically active tissues: brown fat, muscle, and your microbiome—that vast community of microorganisms inhabiting your gut. Each of these prefers a specific type of food for its optimal function. If you don't properly fuel these fat-burning tissues, they aren't going to return the favor by giving you a radical metabolism and a healthy weight.

Another critical missing link concerns the role of the much-maligned omega-6 fats—the pariah of both conventional and alternative health experts. We hear so much these days about ditching omega-6s for omega-3 fats, but as it turns out, high-quality omega-6 fats are the most critical fuel for reigniting sluggish mitochondria—the energy engines in your cells. Essential fats and certain essential amino acids fast-track your metabolism for lasting weight loss, as well as being vital to the nourishment of your cell membranes that surround and protect the mitochondria.

As you will read shortly, the mitochondria are linked to the metabolically active "brown fat" that eats up heavy-duty amounts of glucose and fat for dramatic weight and fat loss, and decreased risk of insulin resistance.

In addition, no disease can be healed if your cell membranes—which direct nutrients in and poisons out—are weak and unstable. *Radical Metabolism* is all about what to eat to rebuild and fortify those lipid- (fat)-based cell membranes, so that toxins are prevented from moving up the chain and gunking up the function of every cell, tissue, and organ in your body, from your brain to your thyroid, gallbladder, liver, kidneys, and skin. This is also where omega-6 fats really shine. True healing requires that we protect ourselves at the source—at the cellular level. Finally, breakthrough research reveals how putting back the missing omega-6s can boost cellular energy, to gain vitality and accelerate fat burn.

But reinstating omega-6s is just one unique aspect of *Radical Metabolism*. Eating "good fats" does you no good if you can't properly digest them. So, this program also introduces the forgotten but powerful role bile plays in the body's slimming systems. Bile is stored in the gallbladder to break down dietary fat and remove toxins from the body. Harvard Medical School research has revealed that subjects with improved bile health showed a remarkable spike in metabolism.

Even more fascinating is a study out of Finland finding that people with decreased bile production are nearly ten times more apt to experience hypothyroidism. With low thyroid on the rise, this provides great hope to the millions of hypothyroid sufferers who experience metabolic slowdown as well as fatigue, dry skin, and constipation. Besides hypothyroidism, studies have also connected poor-quality bile with chronic fatigue, migraines, depression, and autoimmune disorders.

If you no longer have your gallbladder, no problem! Unlike other diets, the Radical Metabolism plan helps you compensate for this to ensure you can fully utilize and digest all those good and essential fats that are your body's preferred fuel. This is a key difference between Radical Metabolism and Paleo, Paleo Plus, and/or Ketogenic diets. I don't want you overloading on fats if you don't have a gallbladder or suffer from poor bile quality (as most weight-loss-resistant individuals do) without nutritional backup, as this can result in weight gain instead of weight loss—as well as decreased energy, gastrointestinal problems, stress on the kidneys, and other issues.

PUTTING IT ALL TOGETHER

As you read, *Radical Metabolism* will probably shake up your long-held beliefs and assumptions about what is healthy, especially when it comes to diet. I sure hope so! I'm not just talking about weight loss—I'm talking about staying energized for life. Let's put the brakes on aging—I'm talking about gaining the tools necessary for dodging age-related illnesses so you won't spend years stuck in the hospital revolving door. If you find the word *radical* a bit intimidating, rest assured that the strategies herein are actually really quite simple and straightforward, designed for easy integration into today's busy lifestyle. *However, these simple strategies produce radical results!*

In the first part of this book, you'll learn the scientific basis for the program before moving on to the protocol itself, so you can understand the rationale. I start by laying out my five Radical Rules to rescue a stalled metabolism, which are foundational to the program. Each of the five must be addressed if you want to reignite your internal cellular energy and fat-burning tissues to fix your broken metabolism. More than 80 percent of readers will feel better after just four days of implementing the basic Radical Rules.

In the second half of the book is the eating program itself. It kicks off with a 4-Day Radical Intensive Cleanse, followed by a 21-Day Radical Reboot—a two-part "cellular makeover" diet designed to jump-start your detox pathways and your metabolic healing. The final section expands the menu with fifty amazing recipes, and provides additional guidance for staying on track for the rest of your life. Here is what you'll learn:

- How to harness the power of omega-6 oils to fuel brown fat to effortlessly stoke your fat-burning fires, while fortifying your cell membranes and ridding your body of toxins
- How bitter foods are key to metabolic healing and digestion; these support your gallbladder health, bile flow, fat breakdown, and better absorption of fat-soluble vitamins for immunity and skin health
- The fabulous foods (herbs, fresh veggies, bitters including watercress, and berries) that will kick your metabolism into overdrive, reboot your gallbladder (or replace what's needed in the form of bile salts if you no longer have your gallbladder), and heal your gut by feeding you "from cell to soul"
- How to optimize your protein and amino acid intake to prevent muscle loss, boost your mitochondria, and reset your "metabolic thermostat"
- How to reduce your exposure to unsuspected toxins that may contaminate some of the foods you love, such as bone broth, chocolate, and green tea
- How to modify your kitchen to steer clear of common food contaminants, such as aluminum and Teflon
- How soups and juices can be combined into a powerful cleanse that rejuvenates and resets your system
- How cleansing beverages, such as refreshing hibiscus and dandelion teas, help clear toxins

- A special section about prebiotic and probiotic foods (jicama/yam bean, miso, sauerkraut, yogurt) to optimize immunity

PRACTICING RADICAL SELF-LOVE

If you are like me, with an over-forty metabolism, it's time to shift it into high gear. Who doesn't want to transform a sluggish system to lose those unwanted pounds, have more energy, and tamp down inflammation? If you've been feeling stuck, you're about to get *unstuck*. What would it be like to actually look forward to seeing your reflection in a full-length mirror? How would this change your life? This is no fantasy—it's what many of my clients report after implementing my program.

Here's what women have experienced on the Radical Metabolism plan:

I am down 15 pounds and I can see a difference on my skin! I have very oily skin, and now it's almost normal. This is my third week and I have been sleeping like a baby.

—Vicky O., age 46

Because I am eating such "clean" foods, my thinking is much clearer. I have been able to tackle writing my blog and implementing daily meditation with ease. My blood sugars that I test every morning have been very good. I've lowered my insulin doses and have a vision that I will be totally off meds in a very short time period, at this rate. Pain levels in my knees are also decreasing, making daily walks much more enjoyable. Daily house chores are not such a chore, as well. . . . As an added bonus, I lost 12 pounds and inches around my waist and buttocks!

—Suzanne K., age 61

I have found a great improvement in my chronic inflammation. Until I got the inflammation under control, exercising for me was a painful process, especially the next day when I really paid for it. Now my joints feel much better and I feel less bloated.

—Marianne F., age 50

[The recipes'] overall taste is very good. I love adding all those bitters to my food . . . all other foods started to taste better and fresher. Sesame, sunflower oils, and ghee are a delight. [I'm] feeling good, energetic, reasonably focused, and calm, despite normal load of work and daily stresses. My total loss in twenty-one days was 8 pounds, and 8.5 inches!

—Marina D., age 54

Because this program deals with all the toxic environmental challenges of our modern world, think of it more as a lifestyle program than a "diet plan." For you to regain your health and maintain it over the long run, these changes will need to be permanent. After all, although there are steps you can take to mitigate the toxins in your home, it's unlikely our overall environmental toxicity problem is going to vanish anytime soon.

Lastly, radical times call for radical changes, but these techniques don't *all* have to be implemented overnight. If you begin to feel overwhelmed, simply slow it down a bit . . . you know, baby steps. Stress is as detrimental to your health as bad fats—so getting stressed out over these changes is counterproductive. Please know that we are here to support you every step of the way, online and otherwise. Be kind to yourself. It's important to recognize and applaud even your smallest accomplishments. If it took ten years for your metabolism to turn against you, you can't expect to completely heal the relationship in less than thirty days. But with a little willingness and determination, you *can* succeed. You can radically improve your metabolism and be on your way to an ageless, radiant you.

Let's get started!

QUIZ: IS YOUR METABOLISM UNDER TOXIC STRESS?

Have you experienced any of the following? If so, your metabolism may be toxic and *Radical Metabolism* is the fix. The more symptoms you have, the more you need *Radical Metabolism*! However, realize that you will still benefit even if you only checked one or two symptoms.

SYMPTOMS	CHECK BOX
Metabolism seems to have slowed since turning forty?	
Type 2 diabetes or prediabetes diagnosis	
Insulin resistance	
Suboptimal lipid profile (higher LDL and triglycerides, lower HDL)	
Elevated blood pressure	
Experienced "menopot" before actual menopause: increased belly fat, higher waist-to-hip ratio	
Hungry nearly all the time	
Increasingly irritable and moody between meals	
Need snacks, such as coffee or biscuits, cakes, sweets, chocolate, throughout the day	
Feel tired at 11 a.m. and 4 p.m.	
Constant middle-of-the-night awakenings	
Food allergies or intolerances, such as to gluten or dairy	
History of gallstones or gallbladder surgery	
Nausea, heartburn, burping, reflux (GERD), gas, bloating, or other digestive symptoms	
GI discomfort after eating fatty foods	
Light-colored stools	
Constipation	
SIBO (small intestinal bacterial overgrowth)	
Autoimmune diseases, such as Hashimoto's thyroiditis, rheumatoid arthritis, or multiple sclerosis	
Lots of pain and inflammation	
Headaches or migraines	
Sciatica-like pains	
Skin problems, such as rosacea, psoriasis, or dry skin	
Hair loss	
Fatigue not relieved by sleep	
Problems detoxing	
Other "orphan" or mystery symptoms that no one can resolve—do you consider yourself a "tough case" for your health-care providers?	

PART ONE

5 RADICAL RULES TO RESCUE YOUR METABOLISM

1 RESCUING A STALLED METABOLISM

> Even miracles take a little time.
>> —Cinderella's Fairy Godmother

IN THIS CHAPTER, YOU'LL LEARN . . .

- Do you have the tell-tale signs of a toxic metabolism?
- Three metabolically active body tissues that influence food cravings and fat storage
- How to keep your cell membranes—the "gatekeepers"—happy
- How an ailing gallbladder can put your slimming in a slump
- The Five Radical Rules for rescuing your metabolism

If you're like most people, you are having more difficulty losing weight as you get older. You may also be experiencing some "mystery symptoms" for which you've not been able to pinpoint a cause—maybe chronic pain, brain fog, or fatigue. How many boxes did you check in the quiz at the end of the Introduction? Perhaps you have just been diagnosed with an autoimmune condition, such as Hashimoto's thyroiditis or rheumatoid arthritis. The latest science reveals seemingly unrelated connections where we previously thought there were none. The effects of a toxic metabolism are progressive and potentially devastating, so what may initially appear as a few extra pounds and diminished energy can develop over time into a *much larger problem*.

SOMEONE LIKE YOU

"Amelia" is a forty-two-year-old working mother of two plagued by weight gain, low thyroid, and persistent pain. Despite eating what she thought was a healthy diet and exercising several days a week, as well as coaching volleyball, she has seen her waistline steadily expand since the birth of her daughter thirteen years ago. She has lost the same 30 pounds three times in the last decade.

Amelia's annual check-ups are unremarkable, except for a slow and steady upward creep of her blood pressure and triglyceride levels. At her last checkup, her triglycerides were up to 175, and her blood pressure (BP) had shot up from 90/60 to 145/85. This rise in BP, along with Amelia's weight gain, have prompted her overzealous doctor to recommend blood pressure medication, but she is reluctant to start down the pharmaceutical path.

A year ago, Amelia had her gallbladder removed after a severe bout with gallstones. Her doctor reassured her she didn't need her gallbladder, that she would be fine without it and feel much better. However, she swears her metabolism took a nosedive after the surgery and her constipation is now worse than ever. Her annoying belly bulge is definitely moving in the wrong direction. Amelia's doc reassures her that she's just having normal "age-related changes" and it's nothing to worry about. Nevertheless, she *does* worry and she is not happy with how her body looks or feels.

Amelia also began having trouble with gastric reflux, which started right after she began a new diet that all her friends raved about. She was doing everything the diet said to do, exactly by the book—eating more "good" fat, going gluten- and dairy-free, cutting out sugar, walking more. Yet she felt terrible, often experiencing abdominal pain and bloating after dinner, with alternating bouts of constipation and diarrhea. Despite being very tired at night, she was not sleeping well. The fatigue was becoming debilitating and she could hardly get through the day. Her relationship with her husband was deteriorating as her interest in sex severely waned, and she was short-tempered with her moody adolescent daughter.

Nothing she tried seemed to make any notable difference. Was this how aging was going to be? After all, many of her friends were reporting the same issues, so *maybe this was normal* . . . what a depressing thought. She began giving in to sugar cravings, which immediately put back on that little bit of weight she'd lost—and then some.

Does this scenario sound familiar?

Amelia is a composite of what I hear every day with my clients. Stubborn weight gain, fatigue, sleep problems, mood swings, digestive issues, lab test values moving in the wrong direction, and the like are typical. Primary care providers often try to reassure their patients that nothing is wrong, which only adds to their patients' frustration. The common denominator is a crashing metabolism—and it's *not* normal and should not be ignored. The good news is, it can be reversed!

What you will read in this chapter gets down to *health on the cellular level*. Weight-loss resistance boils down to damage at the level of the cell, and to cell membranes in particular. Sadly, this is an area that has been ignored in health care, including integrative and functional medicine.

There are three metabolically active tissues that directly relate to how your body uses energy and stores fat. Each of these three tissues requires a different type of fuel and has specific nutritional requirements for optimal function. Unless each is specifically addressed, your slim-down may end up in a shutdown, leading you down the road to metabolic syndrome.

What is metabolic syndrome, exactly? Also referred to as prediabetes, metabolic syndrome is a cluster of symptoms defined as the following: increased blood pressure, elevated blood sugar, increased abdominal body fat, and abnormal lipid or triglyceride levels. When these symptoms occur together, as is often the case, your risk increases for obesity, type 2 diabetes, stroke, and heart disease. Many people with weight-loss resistance also meet the criteria for metabolic syndrome, and insulin resistance is nearly always part of the scene.

Insulin is the hormone responsible for moving sugar into your cells from your bloodstream. *Insulin resistance* means that the various organs and tissues of your body have become resistant to insulin's signals, so more and more insulin is produced. When insulin levels in your blood rise, you tend to gain weight. Conversely, when your insulin levels fall, you tend to lose weight. Insulin resistance leads to chronically elevated blood sugars, which are damaging to the body and can result in type 2 diabetes. This is why many diabetics eventually end up with neuropathy, kidney and blood vessel damage, and pancreatic damage such that insulin can no longer be produced at all.

What's the solution? If your slimming efforts are in a slump, it could be that one or more of the Five Radical Rules to Rescue Metabolism needs to be addressed.

Before we take a deeper dive into the Radical Rules, let's review a few fundamental concepts, starting with metabolism. Then, we'll take a look at the profound role cell membranes play in metabolism, health, and illness. I'll also introduce (briefly) the relatively new science of epigenetics, which has radically transformed our understanding of health and disease. Epigenetics is a concept of how changes occur in the body—such as how your body goes from a healthy state to an unhealthy one, and vice versa. Epigenetics controls your gene expression without changing the genes themselves. And the best news of all is that you are in control of your genes: your genes are not your destiny!

WHAT IS METABOLISM?

Let's start with the basics. The term *metabolism* comes from the Greek word for "change." Your metabolism transforms the food you eat into energy via a kaleidoscope of life-sustaining chemical reactions that mostly occur at the level of the cell. But metabolism affects much more than how many calories you can consume each day without gaining weight—it influences the health of your entire body. We need to broaden our concept of metabolism because it literally controls everything, every biological activity down to each and every cell membrane. Your body has about 37 trillion cells, and not one of them can function well if its membranes are compromised. Even though you're not aware of it, metabolic processes are going on in your body around the clock.

Everything is controlled at the cellular level—appetite, fat burning and fat storage, energy production, hormones, tissue repair, recovery from illness or injury, resistance to disease, and even aging itself. Your metabolism controls digestion, getting nutrients into the cell *and waste products out*. You can thank your metabolism for your body's ability to detoxify itself.

Your diet matters because metabolic processes depend upon the nutrients you eat. These nutrients can be broken down to produce energy and critical proteins, such as DNA. With the assistance of enzymes, metabolic reactions are organized into metabolic pathways that allow basic nutritional components to be transformed into other compounds. A similar process exists for detox pathways.

If you have a weight problem, the difference between you and your friend who seems able to eat anything and never gain an ounce is that she has a more optimized metabolism. Many people have developed what I call a toxic metabolism—which occurs when those critical chemical reactions go awry. Your body depends on certain nutrients to perform those basic functions, and if you can't get them, or for some reason your body can't use them, then systems begin to break down.

It's important to realize that excessive weight gain is just a symptom of a deeper problem—your body's way of clueing you in that something is wrong. And weight gain isn't the only red flag. Maybe your last blood test showed an elevation in your blood glucose or a suboptimal lipid profile. Perhaps your thyroid function was subclinically low. These and many other symptoms are ways your metabolism sends out an SOS—but it's up to you to decipher the signs!

Toxic metabolism means your cells are not getting all the nutrients they need, or your body has a problem with toxicity—*and unfortunately most people have both*. If detox fails, toxins progressively accumulate. Having a toxic body is a bit like swimming in a pool that's never had its water changed.

Not only is the standard American diet (SAD) sorely lacking in nutrition, but toxins are ubiquitous in our environment today. A massive database from the American Chemical Society has logged more than 100 million different chemicals.[1] Are we enjoying "better living through chemistry"? Maybe not! These chemicals are making their way into our foods, our water, and our air, in countless ways—from beef raised under the influence of chemicals and hormones, to plastic bottles infusing water with endocrine-disrupting chemicals. Our bodies perform rather heroically to keep us cleaned out, considering what a monumental task this is.

Toxic metabolism places great stress on the body from increased toxic burden, disrupted hormone signaling, and increased inflammation, which paves the way for obesity and a number of devastating illnesses. One in three seniors now dies with Alzheimer's or another form of dementia, and we have recently learned that this horrible disease may stem directly from a defect in the brain's detoxification system. Heart disease remains the number-one killer of men and women in the United States today, claiming more than 600,000 lives every year—that's one in every four deaths.[2] One in three adults has prediabetes or full-blown type 2 diabetes. Sadly, our children and pets are even showing these trends.

That's the bad news, but here's the good: *Because these diseases share a similar cause, they also share a similar solution.* By correcting toxic metabolism, you can reverse those conditions while at the same time melting off those extra pounds so you'll feel younger, more vibrant and alive than you have in years. The boomerang bulge around your middle will stay away this time because you'll have removed the cause and created what we *all* desire and deserve—*a radical metabolism!*

WHAT WE LEARNED FROM *THE BIGGEST LOSER*

Most traditional diets fail because regaining weight is alarmingly easy. The most profound illustration to date is a 2016 study published in the journal *Obesity* involving fourteen contestants from the weight-loss competition reality show *The Biggest Loser*.[3]

Researchers discovered thirteen of the fourteen contestants had regained at least some of the weight they had lost during the competition, and five were *above* their precompetition weight. Not only had the participants regained an average of 90 pounds/40kg (about 70 percent of their lost weight), but they had a greater appetite and slower metabolism than people of comparable age and body composition who had never lost an extreme amount of weight.

What happened? Researchers discovered that the contestants' leptin level had outright plummeted after the show—and never recovered. Leptin is the satiety hormone that tells you when you've eaten enough. This matches prior reports of former contestants' experiencing uncontrollable hunger and food cravings after the competition.

Although this is the most extreme account, most people regain at least some of the weight they lose from dieting. The more weight you have to lose, the larger your metabolic drop may be—whether you exercise or not. Your body is absolutely relentless in its determination to regain its metabolic set point.

Your weight is determined, at least in part, by a long-standing relationship between energy intake and output. It is controlled by a complex network of hormones.

These hormones exert profound effects in your brain, especially the hypothalamus, which strongly influences your diet and appetite. Think of this as your internal body weight thermostat. How this thermostat works is not well understood, but we do know it is influenced by a multitude of factors, such as activity level, diet, appetite, lifestyle habits, living situation, psychological factors, overall health, and genetics.

When you try to change your weight, your body's natural tendency is to fight back so as to maintain homeostasis, or its set point. It will try to manipulate you into eating more food and oftentimes the wrong food. This explains why it is difficult for most people to maintain a weight that is different from their set point—and the greater the difference, the more the body pushes back.

The bottom line here is that regaining lost weight does not mean you're a failure— you're simply missing a metabolic link! One good piece of news from the *Biggest Loser* study is that more than half of the contestants kept 10 percent of their weight off. But *you* can improve those odds by transforming your toxic metabolism into a radical one. You will now have critical information they didn't have. Metabolism is controlled by hormones, and hormones all operate at the level of the cell membrane. In showdowns between hormones and willpower, hormones always win—until you learn how to outsmart them!

SOLVING PROBLEMS AT THE MICRO LEVEL: CELL MEMBRANE MEDICINE

Someday the area of "membrane medicine" will attain the same popular recognition as probiotics. It's this: You live or die by the health of your cells. They're that important— they're running the show. Your organs and tissues cannot be healthy without your cells, and your cells cannot be healthy without strong cell membranes. *The metabolic magic can only occur if you stay on good terms with these cellular gatekeepers.*

Here's the skinny. It was once thought that cell walls, or membranes, were simply overwraps to hold the cell together, like plastic wrap around a sandwich. But now we know they are complex, ever-changing structures vital to many of the cell's functions. The most basic function of the outer cell membrane is to separate the cell's inside components from its outside environment, providing structural integrity. However, the cell membrane is also the "stage manager," controlling who gets in (nutrients) and who gets out (toxins). The membrane allows certain molecules to enter and exit as needed and must be tough enough to keep out invading organisms. It is constructed essentially of two layers of fat cells.[4]

Besides the outer cell wall (the often-mentioned cell membrane), there are many membranes around components *inside the cell.* Membranes surround the energy-producing mitochondria. There is also a membrane protecting the nucleus of the cell, which contains its genetic material (DNA). The basic structure of all these membranes is the same for your many trillions of cells. Cell membranes make up a significant portion of your body—if you were to lay them all out, the membrane surface area would cover 100 square kilometers. The membrane surface area in your liver alone is equivalent to around five football fields![5]

One reason the fats you eat are so important is that *all* these cell membranes are composed of fat. In fact, cell membranes account for most of the fat in your body. Every cell is composed of three specific types of fat: phospholipids (lipids containing phosphorous), glycolipids (lipids with sugars), and cholesterol. The most important are the phospholipids. Phosphatidylcholine is the most important of those, accounting for half of your cells' total lipid mass.

YOU ARE WHAT YOU EAT—LITERALLY!

There are three ways a cell can be damaged: damage to the outer cell membrane (cell wall), damage to the power supply (mitochondria), and damage to the genetic code (DNA). All involve damage to membranes, which are your cells' first-line defense for protecting the valuables inside. DNA damage is often lethal, resulting in cell mutations or cell death, and this is the mechanism driving autoimmune and degenerative processes, as well as a stalled metabolism.

Cell membranes undergo damage from environmental toxins (mercury, lead, fluoride, etc.), and of course from poor diet. If you eat highly processed fats, your body actually *incorporates them* into your cell membranes, which causes those membranes to deteriorate. This is the ultimate proof that "you are what you eat"—right down to the cellular level! Garbage in, garbage out. We now know that fatty acids modify the actual structure and physical properties of cell membranes, influencing the cellular processes that rely on this structure.

Your membranes can also be damaged by sugar. Actually, any food that triggers an insulin response activates a membrane-destroying enzyme named phospholipase A2. That is why the Radical Metabolism diet eschews all forms of sugar, processed foods, and soft drinks, as well as excessive fruit and grains.

Science has revealed that your body incorporates dietary fatty acids into your cell membranes *within minutes* of digesting them in a process called lipid membrane reorganization. This explains how what you eat is directly involved in various diseases, such as type 2 diabetes, cancer, heart disease, autoimmune and inflammatory disease—even aging itself. If your cells are constructing their membranes from poor-quality fatty acids, such as denatured vegetable oils and trans fats, their ability to transfer oxygen from the bloodstream into the cell will be compromised—and this is an enormous problem. The mitochondria need cellular oxygen (plus fat and sugars) to produce energy, and oxygen in the cell interior is required to prevent disease. In efforts to extend shelf life, typical commercial oils are so overcooked and overprocessed that they *resist oxygen*, rather than attract it. So, if your cells are incorporating these damaged, oxygen-resisting oils into their membranes, then you're in trouble. We will be talking much more about these oils in Chapter 3.

Here's the good news. *If cell membranes can be altered—for better or for worse—in just minutes, imagine what you can accomplish in twenty-five days with the Radical Metabolism plan!*

MIGHT YOU BE RUSTING?

Injury to cell membranes has immediate and severe consequences for all aspects of your body. Because cell membranes are made of fats, they are susceptible to a damaging process called lipid peroxidation, which occurs when free radicals "steal" electrons from the lipids in cell membranes. This is akin to olive oil in your pantry turning rancid. When it happens in your body it has the following effects:

- Increased metabolic toxicity and loss of metabolic "firepower"
- DNA damage
- Poor cell signaling of the immune system
- Disrupted hormone signaling (estrogen, progesterone, testosterone, thyroid, insulin, leptin, etc.)
- Reduced energy production by mitochondria, and mitochondrial diseases (chronic, degenerative, and autoimmune)
- Poor tissue and organ function
- Increased risk of cardiovascular disease
- Increased risk of cancer due to abnormal cell proliferation

Cell membrane damage is intimately linked to both insulin resistance and weight-loss resistance, as your metabolism depends on proper cellular signaling. Think of it as cellular "rust"—the body is unable keep up with repairs from ongoing damage.[6, 7]

How does the body respond to damage? Inflammation. Specifically, *cellular inflammation*. When a cell membrane is inflamed, toxins can't be eliminated and become trapped inside the cell, essentially turning it into a garbage dump, and illness ensues. Inflammation drives cardiovascular disease, cancer, hormone imbalance, diabetes, and so many other conditions that are rampant today. The cells will only be able to function again if they can purge their accumulated toxins, and for this to happen, their membranes must be healed.

YOUR GENES ARE NOT YOUR DESTINY AFTER ALL

There's another amazing function cell membranes perform. Cell membranes can actually turn genes off and on. We used to think our genes controlled our destiny, but the science of epigenetics has turned that model on its head. Our genes are actually malleable!

Simply stated, epigenetics is the study of the changes produced by variations in gene expression, rather than from alterations of the genetic code itself. These changes affect how your cells interpret your genetic blueprint. Think of your DNA as the operating system and your epigenome as the apps—which get updated on a daily or even hourly basis. Epigenetic changes occur when genes are flipped on and off in response to a variety of conditions. These changes are triggered by such factors as diet and lifestyle habits, environmental stimuli, and even thoughts and emotions. Basically, *everything you do* affects your genetic expression—eating, sleeping, exercising, laughing, crying, loving, raging. The field of epigenetics has provided new insights into everything from weight-loss resistance to heart disease to mental health.

We now know that epigenetics can influence how metabolism gets altered, for better or for worse. Take stress, for example. Stress is a huge epigenetic factor. Disease boils down to our ability or inability to adapt to stress. If we don't adapt, we may turn on bad genes. Consider two people who both possess a breast cancer gene. One person has major life stresses but does not learn effective stress management. The other individual has learned to effectively manage her stress. The stressed-out person may have her cancer gene "flipped on," resulting in the manifestation of breast cancer, whereas the unstressed person never manifests it. This is how epigenetic changes occur. The important thing to understand here is, whether we're talking about cancer or weight gain, our genes are continuously being flipped on and off, every moment of the day.

Many describe their weight-loss struggles as feeling like a "switch" has been flipped—a metabolic circuit breaker has been tripped and they can't seem to reset it. And just as with the electricity in your house, everything comes to a halt. Does this describe you? This analogy isn't that far from the truth. When you implement the protocols in this book, what you're really doing is changing your genetic expression, sort of "flipping a switch" to produce healing by actually reprogramming your DNA.

RADICAL METABOLISM TO THE RESCUE

With that in mind, let's move on to my Five Radical Rules to rescue metabolism.

To create a radical metabolism—a fat-fueled metabolism that keeps you lean, healthy, and energized—there are five primary objectives. Each will be covered in detail in the next several chapters, but first let's look at the big picture.

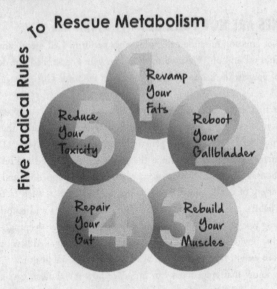

Five Radical Rules To **Rescue Metabolism**

1. Revamp Your Fats
2. Reboot Your Gallbladder
3. Rebuild Your Muscles
4. Repair Your Gut
6. Reduce Your Toxicity

RADICAL RULE #1: REVAMP YOUR FATS

Eating enough omega-6 fat is vitally important to your metabolism and the health of your cell membranes, and it's crucial to eat the right kinds.

When I embarked on my quest to find the cause of toxic metabolism, my first "ah-ha" moment had to do with the pervasive misunderstanding about omega-6 essential fatty acids. Unfortunately, many nutrition and health experts today are demonizing all omega-6s and idolizing all omega-3s. If you learn nothing else from this book, please learn this: *the idea that all omega-6 fats fuel inflammation is a myth!*

While it's true most people in the United States consume far too many omega-6s, they're consuming large quantities of *the toxic variety*—which is completely different than the health-supporting omega-6 fats present in fresh whole foods. We are far too reliant on processed foods, which are simply loaded with overheated, ultrarefined oils. Remember—almost the instant you eat them, your body inserts these chemically adulterated fats into your cell membranes. Toxic omega-6s are indeed pro-inflammatory and deliver none of the health benefits of real omega-6s.

The truth is, we don't consume enough good omega-6s *or* omega-3s, and we eat far too many overheated, oxidized, cell membrane–destroying oils that drive up inflammation and disease. Therefore, the first Radical Rule is to eliminate those adulterated oils and replace them with high-quality omega-6 and omega-3 fats—*in the proper balance*.[8] The optimal ratio of omega-6 to omega-3 is 4:1.

Of course, proper fat metabolism is required for your body to make use of these or any other dietary fats, which brings us to the second Radical Rule: supporting bile and your gallbladder.

RADICAL RULE #2: RESTORE YOUR GALLBLADDER

When it comes to reversing a toxic metabolism and losing stubborn extra body fat, the importance of bile and the gallbladder cannot be overstated. Even though many physicians write off the gallbladder as a "throwaway organ," they are dead wrong. Your gallbladder performs many essential physiological functions that dramatically affect metabolism.

Bile is made in the liver for the purposes of breaking down the fats you eat and escorting toxins out of your body. The gallbladder is a muscular pear-shaped organ located just beneath your liver whose purpose is to store, concentrate, and eject bile when needed. Without an infusion of bile, you can't digest or absorb fat-soluble nutrients, vitamins A, D, E, and K, and those important fat-burning essential fatty acids I just talked about—and as you've already learned, those fats are critical for healthy cell membranes. In addition to cell membranes, fats are also key for brain health, hormone production, immune processes, energy, and cardiovascular health. Your brain is about 60 percent fat and, unlike the rest of your body, does not use fat as its primary source of fuel.

Gallbladder disease and obesity are occurring at epidemic rates. As it turns out, the two are related—*and the connection is bile*. The reason so many people are losing their gallbladder is they've developed thick, sludgy, congested bile that literally mucks up the works. The standard American diet is the perfect setup for toxic bile. Once bile becomes thick, it stops flowing freely into the small intestine and instead stagnates in the gallbladder. Gallstones and inflammation soon follow, and before you know it you're on a gurney headed for the operating room to have your gallbladder removed.

So, what do these gallbladder issues have to do with weight gain? If you can't properly break down fats, they will be absorbed into your bloodstream in an unusable form. Your body has no choice other than to store them—as extra padding on your derriere. An alarming number of people have bile and gallbladder issues but are completely unaware of them. Without healthy bile, you simply can't get those fabulous fat-blasting, immunity-boosting, cell membrane–protecting, fuel-providing benefits— no matter how good your diet is. What you will get is gas, bloating, reflux, constipation, and weight gain.

The time to give your gallbladder some TLC is now because all too often, the first sign of a problem is when the situation becomes critical. There are simple measures for improving gallbladder function and enhancing bile flow, *even if you've had your gallbladder removed*. Chapter 3 will go into this fully, but one key strategy is incorporating more bitter foods into your diet. This includes foods such as watercress, rocket, kale, mustard greens, dandelion greens, grapefruit, ginger, and many others—even dark chocolate.

Many individuals today have an additional problem related to bile quality: insufficient production of stomach acid (hydrochloric acid, or HCl). Without adequate HCl, the release of bile will not be triggered when you eat. Stomach acid deficiency not only compromises digestion of fat but digestion of proteins as well—which brings us to the next Radical Rule.

RADICAL RULE #3: REBUILD YOUR MUSCLES

The third Radical Rule to rescue metabolism is preventing or reversing age-related muscle loss, known as sarcopenia. Guess what accompanies muscle loss—*fat gain!* Although sarcopenia is often characterized as a problem of the elderly, declining muscle mass actually begins much earlier in life and is often accompanied by weight gain, insulin resistance, and metabolic syndrome, which can progress to full-blown type 2 diabetes.[9] *Lean body mass is crucial to your health and longevity.*

If you are sedentary, you can lose 3 to 5 percent of your muscle mass every decade after age thirty. Why do we lose muscle mass as we age? There are several causes, including hormone imbalance, inflammation, lack of movement (especially excess sitting), and inadequate nutrition. Fortunately, *Radical Metabolism* addresses them all.

Two major factors in muscle loss are the consumption of poor-quality proteins and impaired protein digestion. As mentioned in the previous section, many individuals unknowingly suffer from insufficient stomach acid. Protein digestion requires adequate stomach acid and digestive enzymes, and for many of us these are lacking to nonexistent. It's common for people to have a 40 percent decrease in stomach acid production by the time they're in their thirties, and another 50 percent decrease by age seventy. This can lead to such symptoms as gastroesophageal reflux disease (GERD), gas, bloating, nausea and other symptoms (including crankiness). If you are HCl deficient, you will also become mineral deficient because that precious stomach acid is also necessary for mineral absorption. Mineral deficiencies are an enormous issue today.

Amino acids are the building blocks of proteins, so by increasing your consumption of high-quality proteins and amino acids, your body will receive the nutrients it requires to make muscle and other lean body tissues. At the risk of sounding like a recording, amino acids are also critical for building *strong cell membranes*. In Chapter 4, we will look at amino acids in detail, particularly the ten essential amino acids you must consume every day to maintain lean body mass. Like essential fatty acids, there are *essential amino acids*. Your body can't store amino acids as it can carbohydrates and fat, so eating protein daily is imperative.

Of course, no matter how great your diet or supplements, none of this matters if your digestive system itself is unhealthy, so the fourth Radical Rule is to restore the health of your gastrointestinal tract.

RADICAL RULE #4: REPAIR YOUR GUT

Our digestive tract has really taken a beating. Gut inflammation is rampant today, and once the gut is inflamed, the rest of the body soon follows. Individuals with high intestinal permeability ("leaky gut") are much more susceptible to accumulation of abdominal fat, hormone imbalance, metabolic syndrome, and type 2 diabetes. An imbalanced microbiome is directly linked to obesity and weight-loss resistance. Your metabolism is impacted by the overall number of microorganisms living in your digestive tract, as well as their diversity.

Scientists are now realizing the importance of the microbiome, a vast army of health-sustaining microorganisms that populate the gut and are critical to our digestion. They serve as our frontline immune defenses as well. Like the rest of your cells, your microbiome is under attack by environmental toxins, poor diet, parasitic infections, hormone imbalances, antibiotics and other drugs, as well as emotional stress—all of which contribute to dysbiosis. *Dysbiosis*, or an imbalance in gut flora, means you have too few "friendly" microorganisms and too many "unfriendly" ones, which is the perfect storm for local and systemic inflammation.

A wide range of maladies come from dysbiosis, such as leaky gut syndrome, food allergies, small intestine bacterial overgrowth (SIBO), irritable bowel, constipation and diarrhea, fatigue, skin problems, increased toxicity, and all the problems that come from increased toxic body burden—diabetes, heart disease, dementia, arthritis, autoimmune diseases, and the like. Your microbiome also helps control your pH balance and cholesterol levels.

An imbalanced microbiome is also associated with psychological and neurological problems via newly discovered gut-brain connections. Recent science reveals the gut is basically a "second brain" lined with more than 100 million nerve cells that control much more than digestion—they control emotions as well.[10] Ever have the sensation of "butterflies in your stomach," for example? This is your enteric nervous system talking to you.

Several strategies are necessary to restore an ailing gut. First and foremost, repopulating the gut with beneficial flora from probiotic foods, such as naturally fermented sauerkraut and kimchi, as well as optimizing the conditions that support their thriving, such as fiber and prebiotics. Some people do not tolerate probiotic foods and require a modified approach.

RADICAL RULE #5: REDUCE YOUR TOXIC LOAD

The last, but not the least Radical Rule is to reduce your toxic load. If your body has a heavy toxic burden, it cannot function optimally or perform its many metabolic operations. There simply aren't enough resources to go around.

Today we live in a sea of toxins, from the hormone-disrupting chemicals (known as obesogens) in our everyday products that hijack our estrogen receptors, to heavy metals and electropollution that relentlessly assault our DNA. When your body is toxic, all your resources are needed just to keep the poisons cleared out—and this leaves precious few to fire up fat burning. What many people need is a radical cleanup! In Chapters 6 and 7, you will gain tips and strategies for reducing your toxic load— starting in your kitchen. You'll learn where fat-promoting toxins hide, as well as how to best support your body in getting rid of them.

Now that you have the big picture, let's take a closer look at the first Radical Rule— those fabulous fats that are a foundational part of the Radical Metabolism Plan!

2 RADICAL RULE #1: REVAMP YOUR FATS

You gotta nourish to flourish.

—Unknown

IN THIS CHAPTER, YOU'LL LEARN . . .

- The big fat lies that can derail your metabolism
- A radical shift in thinking about omega-6 and omega-3 fats
- The "forbidden fat" you should never stop eating
- The type of body fat you actually want *more* of to help you lose unwanted pounds
- Fats to use and fats to lose to turn your metabolism from fatigued to fantastic

Prepare to have your mind blown—this chapter will free you from fifty years of nutritional fat fallacies that have derailed your metabolism. The first Radical Rule is to revamp the fats in your diet. Eating enough of the right kinds of fat is vitally important to shift your metabolism into fat-burning mode, nourish your cell membranes, and supercharge your energy.

When it comes to how dietary fat influences body fat, there are volumes of half-truths and misunderstandings that have been damaging people's health and waistlines for decades. Good health requires more than good intentions. You need the right information, and so much of what you've been told is simply not true. Let's start with one of the most persistent myths of them all: *eating fat makes you fat.*

It's shocking to me how many people still believe this myth. Despite mountains of evidence to the contrary, it

Myth: Eating fat makes you fat.

continues to be circulated—even by so-called nutritional experts. The latest research is clear: It's not fat that makes us fat; rather, it's refined sugar and toxicity—but that's only the tip of the iceberg. If you still believe that eating fat will make you fat, then read on because, by the time you reach the end of this chapter, I promise you'll be doing your happy dance.

Think about the most popular dietary recommendation from the last fifty years: *low fat, high carbohydrate*. This is exactly *the opposite* of what we should have been eating to optimize our metabolism and health, so it's not surprising that obesity, diabetes, heart disease, and many other illnesses are now raging out of control.

Fears about fat originated way back in the 1950s with a deeply flawed report by researcher Ancel Keys. In his Seven Countries Study, Keys cherry-picked data to support his theory that fat consumption—especially saturated fat—resulted in cardiovascular disease. The media ran with it, and by 1961, even the American Heart Association had issued anti-fat guidelines. What the media got rolling, the food industry delivered with an avalanche of low-fat processed food products claiming to "save us" from those terrible foods that supposedly clogged up our parents' arteries and shortened their lives. Sadly, low-fat, high-carb diets have led millions to an early grave, and to this day, many health experts still cling to these misinformed and rehashed health-damaging recommendations, good intentions notwithstanding.

The truth is, your body cannot make its cells without dietary fat. Your body requires fat for hormone production, cell messaging, and keeping inflammation at bay. Fats are crucial to the function of your heart, brain, and nervous system. Most important, fats are what make up your cell membranes—only now are we beginning to understand the enormity of this fact.

I have been on the front lines of the "fat wars" for decades now. When it comes to cutting-edge science about fats and metabolism, there are a few key players I need to mention for their stellar contributions. Patricia Kane, director of the Neurolipid Research Foundation, is a pioneer in cell membrane science and the importance of essential fatty acids for healthy cell membranes, which she calls "membrane medicine." Another noteworthy individual is Professor Brian Peskin, one of the world's leading authorities on essential fatty acids and their role in the body's metabolic pathways. Peskin coined the term *parent essential oils* (PEOs), which you will be learning about shortly. Another scientist of note is Aaron Cypress, MD, PhD, MMSc, of the National Institutes of Health. Dr. Cypress published groundbreaking new information about the thermogenic properties of brown fat. There are others as well whose great work provides the foundation for the concepts presented in *Radical Metabolism*.

Before we dive into the importance of fats for cell membranes, we need to understand some basic information about your body's fuel preferences.

YOUR BODY WAS BUILT TO RUN ON FAT—NOT SUGAR!

One key goal for turning a sluggish metabolism into a radical one is to shift your body from sugar-burning mode into fat-burning mode. You can't do this if you're skimping on dietary fats. While supplying your body with those metabolism-boosting fats, you must also reduce your sugar consumption, as well as carbohydrates that your body converts into sugar.

The human body is amazing in its ability to run on different types of fuel—specifically, sugar and fat. Fat is the optimal fuel for humans—*our body was* not *meant to use glucose (sugar) as a primary fuel source.*

Today, the typical diet is so high in sugar and carbs, people's metabolic engines are stuck in glucose-burning mode because of its constant supply. This was not the case with our hunter-gatherer ancestors whose diet was very low in sugar, so their body had to rely on fat stores for fuel. Like an unused muscle, our fat-burning engines have weakened and in some cases completely shut down.

A sugar-fueled metabolism creates a number of problems. It causes your blood glucose and insulin levels to spike and leads to more sugar and carb cravings, overeating, and increased storage of body fat—especially belly fat, also known as visceral fat. Fat around your visceral organs—such as your liver, pancreas, and intestines—produces more inflammation and insulin resistance than does the fat under your skin (subcutaneous fat). Burning glucose instead of fat generates more free radicals in your body, leading to increased oxidative damage and inflammation. Cancer cells also thrive on sugar.

Studies now tell us that artificial calorie-dense forms of another sugar, fructose (such as the glucose-fructose syrup/high-fructose corn syrup that's loaded into soft drinks and processed foods) are particularly damaging to your metabolism and overall health. High fructose consumption increases your risk for metabolic syndrome, obesity, type 2 diabetes, cardiovascular disease, and nonalcoholic fatty liver disease (NAFLD).[1] Incredibly, about 30 percent of the general population and 70 percent of obese individuals have NAFLD.[2] Why? Your liver immediately converts fructose into fat! Even worse, it leaves behind a trail of toxic metabolites (uric acid, for one)—much like those generated from the metabolism of alcohol.

The good news is, by shifting your diet you can shift your body's metabolic engine from sugar-burning to fat-burning mode. You need *some* dietary sugar, but once your fat-burning engines are reignited, that requirement is minimal. A fat-burning metabolism is more efficient: it stabilizes your blood sugar and insulin levels, reduces cravings, melts off body fat, starves cancer cells, and quells inflammation.

Increasing fats and decreasing sugars is a principle common to other diets, such as Paleo and Ketogenic, but there's a problem. *Many individuals have difficulty digesting and metabolizing fats.* If you don't address this issue, then simply eating more healthy fats and less sugar is not going to result in the metabolic shift and weight loss you're looking for—and you may even get sick. You must go a step further and optimize your body's ability to actually use those fats. This is what this program does—it goes beyond Paleo and Keto and what you end up with is a lean machine . . . *a radical metabolism*!

MEMBRANE MEDICINE

Healing your metabolism starts at the level of the cell. The intelligence of a cell lies in its membrane, even more than its nucleus. The nucleus houses DNA, but that's about all. It has all the data but initiates none of the activity—functioning more like a library. On the other hand, the cell membrane uses the DNA for reference and then tells it what to do, directing all cellular activities. Biologist and epigenetics scientist Bruce Lipton, PhD, dubbed these amazing cellular structures "mem-Brains."

Those little mem-Brains are embedded with thousands of hormone receptors. Hormones direct cellular function, but it's the cell's *receptors* that are responsible for "hearing" those hormone messages. Most of today's rampant endocrine problems are the result of damaged hormone receptors—therefore, the answer lies in repairing these receptors. But instead, what is typically done is to throw more hormones at the system, which does nothing to fix the problem and actually makes receptors tune out even more. This is called hormone resistance.

One type of hormone resistance involving the metabolism is insulin resistance, which if not addressed may lead to type 2 diabetes. Insulin, made in the pancreas, is the hormone that controls blood glucose levels and storage. Type 2 diabetics have plenty of insulin, but their insulin receptors have gone deaf. *The way to reverse hormone resistance is to mend the cell membranes—fixing the problem at its source.*[3]

Proper dietary fats make membranes more fluid and efficient. Toxins also tend to attach to cell membranes, and fortunately the same membrane-stabilizing diet helps remove them. Hormone receptors are attached and stabilized by little structures called lipid rafts, which become damaged by inflammation. Lipid rafts are made of saturated fat and cholesterol—*so these two fats can literally heal your hormones.*

Speaking of cholesterol, the latest studies have confirmed there is no connection between the consumption of saturated fats and increased risk for heart disease, or between cholesterol and heart disease. You can finally stop worrying about eating cholesterol-rich foods and saturated fats (as long as they're of the nutritious variety, such as eggs and grass-fed meats) because those dietary elements are immensely important to your cell membranes, hormone function, and metabolism.[4]

> The major diseases of our time can be prevented by focusing on the removal of epigenetic toxins and stabilizing cell membranes . . .
> —Dr. Patricia Kane

A key to all these hormone problems—be they insulin, thyroid, or menopause related—is to rebalance and revamp the fats in your diet. That is what makes the Radical Metabolism plan different and why so many other programs fail. If your cells are not getting what they need, they will not function properly. Fix the cell and you fix the problem.

THE CONNECTION BETWEEN INFLAMMATION AND WEIGHT-LOSS RESISTANCE

If you want to have a skinny metabolism, reducing chronic inflammation is absolutely critical, and the Radical Metabolism diet does just that. Inflammation can lead to weight gain as well as numerous illnesses. One of the underlying causes of inflammation is an imbalance in your essential fatty acid intake.

It's important to realize that inflammation itself is not a bad thing—it's only a problem when it rages out of control. Inflammation is your body's way of protecting you—without it, you would never heal from a cut, fight off a cold, or mend a broken leg. When you are injured or threatened with an infection, your immune system sounds the alarm and sends out substances called inflammatory mediators, such as histamine, prostaglandins, and cytokines, to increase blood flow and get specific immune cells to the site of the injury. This is necessary for your body to heal. Acute inflammation can create temporary redness, pain, swelling, and/or fever, but normally this goes away in a day or two. On the other hand, when your body stays perpetually inflamed over time, you can become quite ill.

Chronic inflammation means your immune system is staying activated, and this creates a cascade of unwanted effects in your body, including elevated insulin, among other things. Inflammation makes chemical signals go awry. Your body is under stress so it begins building up its fat reserves. Not only are fat cells little energy warehouses, but they also send out signals that keep the immune system in overdrive. Higher inflammation means more fat cells, and more fat cells lead to higher inflammation—it's a vicious cycle! Spare tires stack up around your middle. Studies show that as your weight increases, so does inflammation.[5]

One of your body's requirements for preventing chronic inflammation, and the weight gain that often accompanies it, is a balanced omega-6 and omega-3 fat intake.

Note: Before we get into how these magical omegas do their thing, I want you to be aware of a resource I've provided for you in Appendix 1. It is a glossary of "lipid lingo" to help you in case you come across any unfamiliar terms. There are many types and classifications of fats, and the terminology can be a bit overwhelming.

OMEGA-6 FATS: THE "FORBIDDEN" FAT
YOU SHOULD NEVER STOP EATING

Lately, a good deal of debate has surrounded omega-3 and omega-6 fatty acids in terms of their biological roles and how much we should be eating. Omega-3s and omega-6s are essential fatty acids (EFAs), meaning they are just that—*essential*. Our body cannot make them, so we must get them from the foods we eat. Omega-3s and omega-6s are both integral parts of the structure and function of cell membranes.[6]

When the scientific community began recognizing inflammation as a major driver of chronic disease, they began to search for the cause. Blood levels revealed most of our diets are extremely top-heavy in omega-6 fatty acids, and light on the omega-3s—so the omega-6s, as a category, were blamed for inflammation, especially arachidonic acid (AA). Omega-6 fats were labeled "pro-inflammatory" and omega-3s as "anti-inflammatory," and the misguided mantra to simply reduce your dietary omega-6s and increase your omega-3s (e.g. supplement with fish oil) spread like wildfire.[7]

The problem is, this is oversimplified. Not all omega-6 fats are equal. It's true that people are overloaded in omega-6, but the type of omega-6 they're overloaded with is the toxic kind, mainly oils destroyed by overprocessing. We're talking about those found in French fries, packaged cookies (made with shortening), and junk food loaded with sugar and hydrogenated vegetable oils—all of which are indeed pro-inflammatory. The increased consumption of hydrogenated vegetable oils represents the single largest increase in any type of food over the last century. One estimate is that Americans now consume 100,000 times more vegetable oils than they did in the year 1900.[8]

Unfortunately, like a bad game of Chinese whispers, the toxicity of junk omega-6 oils became generalized to *all* omega-6s. The truth is that there are also *high-quality functional* omega-6 fats, and we don't get enough of these, nor do we consume enough omega-3s. We are actually deficient in both!

The pervasive recommendation to avoid omega-6 fats is actually counterproductive to your health, metabolism, and weight-loss efforts. Reducing the "good" omega-6s in your diet will only further expand an already-expanding waistline because, as it turns out, functional omega-6s are some of the most powerful fats for activating your fat-burning engines. They have positive benefits for the checks and balances of your body's inflammation system. These omega-6s are extremely restorative to cell membranes, and strong cell membranes are key to achieving proper body weight and a radical

> *Myth: All omega-6 fats are pro-inflammatory, so you need to avoid them all.*

metabolism. We'll talk more about them in the upcoming section "Parent Essential Oils" (page 25).

THE RIGHT RATIO

Thanks to an overabundance of refined vegetable oils, processed foods, grains and grain-fed meats, the standard American diet (SAD) has dramatically thrown our natural essential fatty acid ratio out of balance. *For optimal metabolism, it's important to consume omega-6 and omega-3 fatty acids in the right balance: There seems to be a golden ratio of about 4:1.*

Historically, traditional diets have provided omega-6–to–omega-3 ratios in the range of 1:1 to 5:1, but the standard American diet has us around 20:1. If you have twenty times as many omega-6s as omega-3s, then they are coming from junk oils—meaning they're damaged and provide no nutritional benefit. Adding to the problem is that all those junk omega-6s shut down the omega-3s through a mechanism called competitive inhibition. The omega-3s cannot compete with all those omega-6s, and so the junk omega-6s become incorporated into your cell membranes, weakening them and generating all sorts of problems. Remember—garbage in, garbage out.

It may be a challenge to wrap your head around, but again, it's important to understand that you can be omega-6 dominant *and* have an omega-6 deficiency, at the same time—*your deficiency is in the healthy, functional omega-6s.*

Surprisingly, *most of our cells prefer the omega-6s over the omega-3s—especially our mitochondria, which use omega-6s almost exclusively.* One of the reasons for this is the tendency for the omega-3 fatty acids to oxidize. Oxidized fatty acids are as toxic to your cells as rancid fish oil is objectionable to your nose, causing inflammation and accelerated aging.

Health abnormalities appear more quickly when people are omega-6 deficient versus omega-3 deficient (apart from abnormalities of the heart, brain, retina, and platelets). And when animals are deprived of both omega-3 and omega-6 fatty acids, abnormalities can be corrected with the omega-6s alone, whereas efforts to correct with only omega-3s make many conditions worse. Omega-3s represent about 14 percent of the total lipids in your brain and nervous system (in the form of EPA and DHA), but the omega-6s make up about 10 percent (in the form of arachidonic acid). It follows that *both* must be replenished on a regular basis.

Myth: You need to consume as many omega-3 fatty acids as possible.

YES, YOU CAN TAKE TOO MUCH FISH OIL

You have undoubtedly heard about the benefits of fish oil. Maybe you even take it every day. These benefits exist courtesy of its high omega-3 content. In a study published in *American Journal of Clinical Nutrition*, those who consumed fish oil and walked for forty-five minutes three times per week lost up to 5 pounds more than did the control group, including significant loss of body fat.[9]

The problem is, due to the modern fish oil fervor, many health-conscious individuals have swung the pendulum too far *in the opposite direction*. They've begun taking huge amounts of fish oil or krill oil without balancing it out with functional omega-6s. When omega-3s and omega-6s are in balance all systems are go, but when one overwhelms the other, you get problems.

The omega-3s compete with the omega-6s for incorporation into cell membranes. Studies show that in the omega-3 dominant state (which can occur when supplementing with fish oil alone), omega-3 fatty acids can replace an important fat in the mitochondrial membrane called cardiolipin. Remember, your mitochondria prefer lots and lots of omega-6s. Decreased cardiolipin can cause sudden drops in cellular energy. Mitochondrial illnesses are rampant today, involving nearly every organ system. Because your cells' mitochondria are responsible for producing more than 90 percent of your energy, they are a factor in everything from Alzheimer's to diabetes, degenerative disorders, autoimmunity, certain cancers, and more.[10]

The bottom line is, don't go overboard! Fish oil supplements can be a healthy part of your diet, provided they are balanced out with plant-based omega-3s and omega-6s. To support your metabolism rather than snuff it out, make sure your fish oil is fresh, clean, and unoxidized. Aim for that perfect 4:1 ratio of omega-6s to omega-3s and you'll reap the benefits of both!

POWERFUL FATS THAT FIRE UP YOUR METABOLISM

Now that you understand the reason for a balanced intake of omega-6s and omega-3s, let's start looking at which fats to eat versus which to banish from your dinner plate. We want only the friendly fats that will fire up our fat-burning engines and put us on the fast-track to weight loss, right? Although we'll be incorporating foods high in omega-3s and omega-6s, the "slimming sixes" is a primary focus of the Radical Metabolism plan. First, we will introduce the concept of parent essential oils, and then we'll delve into the all-star players: linoleic acid (LA), alpha-linolenic acid (ALA), gamma-linolenic acid (GLA), and conjugated linoleic acid (CLA).

PARENT ESSENTIAL OILS

When we talk about functional omega-6s and omega-3s, what we're really talking about is pure, non-heated, unprocessed, organic, non-genetically modified oils with all of their natural nutritional benefits intact. As noted earlier, Dr. Brian Peskin coined a term for these oils: parent essential oils (PEOs). There are only two types of PEOs, one omega-6 and one omega-3, respectively: linoleic acid and alpha-linolenic acid.[11] Your body can manufacture several other fatty acids from these two "parent" oils, which is why it's so important to get enough of them in your diet. Professor Peskin argues—and I agree—that damaged (non-functional) essential fatty acids are not desirable, are much less "*essential*," and have no place in our diet.

PEOs are the bricks and mortar of your cells, tissues, and organs, as well as manna for your mitochondria. PEOs also form the foundation of our sex hormones and are known to have a "calming effect" on the endocrine system. Men seem to have a greater PEO requirement than do women. Every cell is 25 to 33 percent PEOs. In general, nuts and seeds and their cold-pressed oils are the primary PEO sources.

LINOLEIC ACID: THE GRAND PUFA FOR METABOLISM

You can think of linoleic acid (LA) as the "PEO CEO"! An omega-6 superstar, linoleic acid is the most powerful parent oil, performing many crucial biological functions. LA is also the most important polyunsaturated fatty acid (PUFA) and is most abundant in seeds, seed oils, and nuts (sunflower seeds, hemp seeds, sesame seeds, high-linoleic sunflower oil and high-linoleic safflower oil, pine nuts, walnuts, and others). Eating these foods is a must for creating a radical metabolism.

Linoleic acid is a key player in the following biochemical processes, which are all involved in your metabolism:

- Maintenance of cell membrane structure
- Enhancing permeability of membranes, including membranes in the skin, digestive tract, and blood-brain barrier
- Prevention of toxins from entering the cell
- Cholesterol transport and synthesis
- Synthesis of eicosanoids (highly important signaling molecules involved in many cellular activities)

A significant portion of the LA you consume is used immediately to maintain and repair inner and outer cell membranes. In fact, a 2009 advisory by the American Heart Association found LA to be cardioprotective.[12] Evidence is mounting that LA, despite being an omega-6 fat, actually has powerful *anti*-inflammatory properties, and is "heart healthy." This is significant because, for so long, the omega-6s have been misunderstood, accused of being pro-inflammatory and therefore increasing your heart attack risk. According to the *New England Journal of Medicine*, diets high in polyunsaturated fat are more effective at stabilizing cholesterol and lowering heart disease risk than are low-fat or high-carb diets.[13] Remember, the benefits we are talking about are from fully functional, unadulterated omega-6 oils, *not* junk oils (such as from corn oil, canola oil (vegetable oil), cottonseed oil, margarine, shortening, etc.) Junk oils will only raise your cardiac risk.[14]

In addition, linoleic acid is an oxygen magnet. For cells to stay healthy, they need high enough oxygen levels for cellular respiration and growth. If cells become oxygen deprived, they malfunction and die. The relationship between linoleic acid and cellular oxygen was underscored by a study in the journal *Pediatrics* involving cystic fibrosis patients.[15] Many of their symptoms were found to result from decreased oxygenation related to LA deficiency.

Where to Get It: Hemp seeds and hemp oil, sunflower seeds and oil, sesame seeds and oil, pine nuts and oil, walnuts, pecans, Brazil nuts, grass-pastured dairy.

ALPHA-LINOLENIC ACID: THE ENERGY-BOOSTING OMEGA-3 PARENT ESSENTIAL OIL

Alpha-linolenic acid (ALA) is the omega-3 PEO. Our body is designed to break down ALA into EPA and DHA, although some individuals may struggle with this conversion. EPA and DHA are the two omega-3s for which fish oils are known. Alpha-linolenic acid comes mostly from plants, with the highest levels found in flaxseed, chia seed, and pumpkin seed oils.

As much as 85 percent of the ALA you consume is used immediately for energy, and the remainder is used to build cell membranes, especially those in your heart, brain, and retinas. Alpha-linolenic acid has demonstrated benefits for your cardiovascular and respiratory systems and is helpful for autoimmune conditions, such as lupus and rheumatoid arthritis. This valuable omega-3 is the starting point for hormone synthesis and is involved in gene expression. There is also evidence that ALA may inhibit the proliferation of estrogen-positive breast cancer cells.[16]

Where to Get It: Flaxseeds and flaxseed oil, chia seeds and chia seed oil, pumpkin seeds and pumpkin seed oil, clary sage oil, sacha inchi seeds, walnuts and walnut oil, Brazil nuts, cashews, hazelnuts, leafy green vegetables, butternut squash, Brussels sprouts, kale, watercress, algae oil.

GLA: THE FAT BURNER OF THE OMEGA-6 KINGDOM

One special omega-6 with profound metabolic implications is gamma-linolenic acid (GLA). This special polyunsaturated fatty acid is unparalleled in promoting fat burning by activating your brown fat. What is brown fat? It is a type of mitochondria-rich adipose tissue often dormant in overweight people. Let me explain.

There are essentially two kinds of fat cells in your body: brown fat and white fat. White fat is the insulating fat layer under your skin that stores excess calories. Brown fat is the special fat-burning tissue that burns excess calories for heat rather than energy. *In other words, brown fat is metabolically active.*

Babies are born with a large amount of brown fat, which helps maintain their body temperature. Animals depend on brown fat to keep them warm during hibernation. Brown fat is located deeper in your body than white fat, surrounding your heart, kidneys, adrenal glands, neck, spine and major blood vessels. The brown color is caused by the presence of concentrated fat-burning cellular units called mitochondria.

Although brown fat composes 10 percent or less of your total body fat, it burns one fourth of all the calories burned by your other fat tissues combined. When activated, brown fat consumes a large quantity of glucose from your bloodstream, helping to keep your blood sugar levels nice and low. Another difference between white and brown fat is that white fat produces pro-inflammatory factors but brown fat generates anti-inflammatory ones. Inflammation often leads to weight gain and further metabolic slowdown.[17]

As we age, we tend to lose brown fat. The more white fat we accumulate, the less metabolically active our brown fat becomes. Thin individuals simply have more "activated" brown fat than do overweight individuals. The good news is that you can reactivate your brown fat if you know the right tricks!

GLA is a brown fat reactivator, giving your mitochondria a boost and causing your body to burn, rather than store, more energy. GLA stimulates a metabolic process commonly referred to as the sodium pump, which helps use up nearly half your body's calories. GLA also induces feelings of fullness by raising serotonin levels. This mighty omega-6 has been found to reduce inflammation, lower blood pressure, quiet PMS, and possibly slow the spread of certain drug-resistant cancers. A steady supply of GLA helps skin retain its moisture to stay supple and smooth.

GLA is a rarely acknowledged rock star when it comes to losing weight, *but nearly everyone is deficient*—even the most health-conscious individuals. Many factors interfere with the body's ability to convert LA into GLA, such as overeating, excess consumption of sugar and refined grains, insulin resistance, thyroid or pituitary problems, vegan diets, protein and vitamin deficiencies, stress, and others. Our ability to make this biological conversion also decreases with age.

Where to Get It: Fortunately, you can get GLA from seed oils, such as blackcurrant seed oil (17 percent), evening primrose oil (10 percent), hemp seeds, and acai berries. I recommend blackcurrant as a supplement because it has the best nutritional balance. If you're stuck in your weight-loss efforts, adding hemp seeds and hemp oil to your diet—and possibly a GLA supplement—may be just the ticket to get things moving again!

CONJUGATED LINOLEIC ACID (CLA)

Conjugated Linoleic acid (CLA) is a critical omega-6 fatty acid that is especially good at shuttling fat away from your belly. CLA is a derivative of linoleic acid found to inhibit an enzyme called lipoprotein lipase, which is involved in the storage of fat in fat cells. Hundreds of CLA studies have been done and not all agree about CLA's benefits. However, there is a substantial body of evidence that CLA may do the following:

- Reduce belly fat, independent of food intake
- Activate brown fat
- Activate thermogenesis
- Increase mitochondrial density in white fat
- Preserve lean body mass
- Reduce appetite
- Balance leptin (the satiety hormone)
- Help prevent osteoporosis
- Reduce inflammation
- Inhibit growth of cancer cells (breast, colorectal, lung, skin, stomach)

Some studies have shown remarkable success with CLA. A group of overweight men lost mostly belly fat and reduced their waistline by 1 inch without making any diet or lifestyle changes.[18] In a similar study, women taking CLA lost mostly belly and thigh fat and reduced their waistline by 1.2 inches. That said, it's always best to get as much of your CLA from whole foods as you can, as opposed to relying exclusively on supplements.

Where to Get It: CLA is found mostly in animal products, highest from grass-pastured. White button mushrooms and pomegranate seed oil are good vegan sources. It's difficult to get therapeutic levels of CLA from foods alone (see the following table), so if you do opt for a supplement, I suggest dosing at 3 to 4 grams per day. One study found 3.2 grams effective for fat loss.

SUPERCHARGE YOUR METABOLISM: IN WITH GOOD FATS—AND OUT WITH THE BAD

Now that you understand the value of parent oils and how they can stoke your metabolic fires, let's look at the foods you can eat to obtain them, as well as foods to avoid.

CLA CONTENT IN FOODS

FOOD	CLA (MG)
Safflower oil	3 mg per tablespoon
Sunflower oil	2 mg per tablespoon
Beef (conventionally raised)	71 mg per 115g
Beef (raised on grass pastures)	433 mg per 115g
Cow's milk (conventionally raised cows)	44 mg per 240ml
Cow's milk (raised on grass pastures)	160–240 mg per 240ml
Cheese (raised on grass pastures)	180–270 mg per 30g
Butter	54 mg per tablespoon
Egg yolk (one large)	3 mg

The following are the most important Do Eats and Don't Eats. Overall, think: fresh whole foods, unprocessed, and as close to the earth as possible. You will find more information and comprehensive food lists in Chapter 9, which details the full Radical Metabolism program.

DO EAT: NUTS

If you're nuts about nuts, then I have great news for you! Nuts (and seeds) are a core part of the Radical Metabolism plan. Nuts have been praised for their nutritional value, but you've been fooled about which nutrients make them so good for us. Their nutritional prowess comes from those mighty *omega-6s*. Even walnuts, long touted as "heart healthy" for their omega-3 content, have *five times as many omega-6s as omega-3s*. It's the omega-6s that actually account for most of their cardiovascular benefits.[19]

Organic almonds, Brazil nuts, pistachios, hazelnuts, pine nuts, and the like are fabulous sources of omega-6 PEOs, but just don't go overboard on them. Make sure they are balanced out with some good omega-3s because competitive inhibition goes both ways. (Note: Choose almonds from Spain because the American variety are irradiated.) Siberian pine nut oil is rich in pinoleic acid (similar to linoleic) and is an excellent remedy for all inflammatory gastrointestinal conditions.

Macadamia nuts are a special case because they have a unique monounsaturated fatty acid called omega-7. Many people have never even heard of this omega. One specific omega-7, palmitoleic acid, is a dynamo when it comes to battling the bulge. This omega-7 has been shown to reduce insulin resistance, lower blood sugar, suppress fat storage, reduce LDL, raise HDL, and be a powerful suppressor of inflammation.[20] It even helps build collagen.[21] So, where do you find this metabolic miracle? Macadamia nuts and oil, sea buckthorn, and deep sea anchovies are the sources.

DO EAT: SEEDS AND COLD-PRESSED SEED OILS

We've already covered how important seeds and seed oils are for providing those glorious parent oils that strengthen cell membranes, optimize hormones, and power up your new body-slimming system. Hemp oil is a metabolic rock star with its 3:1 omega ratio—you can't get much better than that! Hempseeds are 60 percent linoleic acid. Other great omega-6-rich seeds are chia, sunflower, safflower, sesame, flax, pumpkin, and apricot seeds. In addition to being rich in omega-6, apricot kernels are a source of vitamin B_{17} (amygdalin or laetrile), a potential cancer-fighter. Be careful not to overdo the apricot kernels due to their potentially toxic cyanide content.

One of the newer kids on the block is black cumin seed (and its oil), also called black coriander or simply black seed. Black seed comes from the *Nigella sativa* plant, native to Asia, and has powerful healing qualities, including regenerating pancreatic cells in those with diabetes and killing MRSA, a dangerous antibiotic-resistant strain of *Staphylococcus aureus* bacteria. Sacha inchi seeds from Peru, otherwise known as Incan peanuts, are simply loaded with omega-3 and omega-6 fats and protein.

HEMP, HEMP, HOORAY!

Hemp seeds are one of nature's greatest gifts, perfect little bundles of benefits for your entire body. You can reap the hemp's benefits by consuming the oil, seeds (typically these are "hemp hearts" which have had their hulls removed), or by blending them into hemp milk. Hemp seeds are about one third healthful fats and one quarter protein, as well as a magnificent source of natural GLA (gamma-linolenic acid). It's hard to find a food with a better essential fat profile—hemp boasts a 3:1 omega-6-to-omega-3 ratio.

Hemp seeds are also not shy when it comes to protein—equal to beef or lamb but in a more digestible, bioavailable form. They are also a complete protein, providing all of the essential amino acids. Just 30 grams of hemp seeds (2 to 3 tablespoons) contain 11 grams of protein. The fiber in hemp seeds is contained mostly in the hull, so hemp hearts have relatively little fiber. However, what they lack in fiber they make up for in nutrients: calcium, magnesium, iron, manganese, phosphorous, potassium, zinc, and vitamins A, B_1, B_2, B_3, B_6, D, and E. Hemp also has strong anti-inflammatory benefits, most likely related to its abundant GLA.

Overall, these little dynamos can sustain energy, encourage weight loss, reduce food cravings, lower blood pressure, improve blood sugar and lipid profiles, and tamp down inflammation. Hemp hearts have a delightfully delicate nutty flavor and taste good as a topping on salads, veggies, and many other dishes. Consume hemp seeds or hemp oil raw to preserve the delicate fats, and store them in an airtight container in the refrigerator, or freezer.

Hemp belongs to the genus *Cannabis sativa*, cultivated for thousands of years for everything from nutrient-rich seeds and oils to industrial fiber, paper, textiles, building materials, and even fuel. Until recently, the nutritional benefits of hemp were all but ignored due to hemp's being a cousin to marijuana. The truth is that hemp seeds are incapable of producing a "high" because their THC content is so minuscule.

DO EAT: COCONUT OIL AND MCTS

Coconut oil is not an essential fatty acid like your omega-6s and omega-3s. Still, coconut and coconut oil have oodles of brain- and metabolism-boosting benefits, as well as supporting your immune system. About 80 percent of coconut meat is fat, and of that 92 percent is saturated fat. (For those who remember when coconut oil was a "bad guy," keep in mind that the natural, unrefined varieties available in nutrition stores today are vastly different from the ultrarefined, deodorized, and bleached coconut oil added to junk food in the 1980s—which was a cardiovascular nightmare. When we talk about the benefits of coconut oil, we are definitely not talking about those!)

Populations for whom coconut is a dietary staple have much lower rates of cardiovascular and brain disease than do Westerners. Coconuts and coconut oil may offer protection against brain disorders, such as epilepsy and Alzheimer's disease. In a 2015 study, Alzheimer's patients given a daily dose of extra-virgin coconut oil showed significantly improved cognition.[22]

Coconut oil is about two thirds medium-chain fatty acids (MCFAs), also known as medium-chain triglycerides (MCTs). MCTs are far less common than long-chain triglycerides. LCTs (12 to 18 carbons long) are the predominant form of fat in the standard American diet. MCTs (6 to 10 carbons long) are metabolized by the body more like carbohydrates, but they provide energy without any of the insulin-related problems of carbohydrates. They go straight to your liver, where they are turned into ketones and used immediately for energy. MCTs suppress appetite, stabilize blood sugar, raise HDL, and improve overall lipid profile, while encouraging the shedding of excess body fat, especially visceral fat. MCTs also have appetite-suppressing effects.[23] Ketogenic diets are known to be beneficial for certain types of cancer.

Coconut contains a wealth of antioxidants and can be regarded as an antiaging food. It boosts thyroid function, improves digestion and absorption of fat-soluble vitamins, and promotes conversion of cholesterol into pregnenolone, a precursor to many important hormones. Fifty percent of the fat in coconuts is lauric acid, a type rarely found in nature. Your body converts lauric acid into monolaurin, which is a gift to your immune system for its antiviral, antibacterial, antifungal, and antiparasitic properties.

Note: Despite all its health benefits, you will be abstaining from coconut oil during the 4-Day Radical Intensive Cleanse and the 21-Day Radical Reboot, to rebuild your healthy omega-6 and omega-3 fat stores. Then, afterward, once you're on the Maintenance phase of the Reboot, you'll be adding coconut and other healthy fats back again.

DO EAT: OLIVE OIL

Olive oil is not the heart-health panacea that the food industry would have you believe, but in moderation, a high-quality one can be part of a healthy diet. Olive oil is high in oleic acid and is classified as a monounsaturated fatty acid (MUFA). It's in the same category as coconut oil—they are both nonbioactive oils that don't provide much in the way of omega-3s or omega-6s, but they do have other virtues. Olive oil's biggest health asset is its high polyphenol content, which probably accounts for most of its benefits. Polyphenols are micronutrients possessing an abundance of antioxidant properties that do everything from fighting cancer and heart disease to putting the brakes on aging. Olive oil has been shown to help prevent accumulation of visceral fat, even if overall body weight remains unchanged.[24]

Be careful, however—most commercial olive oil products today are so oxidized that precious few nutrients remain. Fake olive oils are also a widespread problem. As much as 80 percent of so-called Italian olive oil is fake, cut with inferior oils, coloring agents, and worse. The industry is riddled with fraud, so you must be extremely careful about your sources.[25]

DO EAT: GRASS-PASTURED ANIMAL PRODUCTS, DAIRY, AND WILD COLD-WATER FISH

Animal products (meat, poultry, eggs, dairy) from animals raised on pasture—eating a biologically appropriate diet of grasses—have been shown to be far more nutritious than conventionally raised meats, where the animals are raised in confined quarters and fed processed food diets consisting of grains and growth-promoting drugs. Three decades of research on grass-pastured meats show superior fatty acid and antioxidant profiles, including higher levels of CLA, minerals, vitamins (including A, B_1 and B_2, and E), and glutathione.[26] Raising livestock that is free to roam on pasture is also more humane and earth-friendly. Conventional animal products contain more bacterial contamination (*Salmonella, Enterococcus, Staphylococcus,* and *E. coli*) due to overcrowding and other industrial practices. Make sure your dairy is full-fat because the fat is where you get those amazing omegas!

Eat fish that are wild-caught from cold waters, and steer clear of farmed fish. Salmon is one of nature's richest sources of omega-3 fatty acids, but make sure you are eating the right kind. Due primarily to their diet, farm-raised salmon have higher concentrations of thirteen pollutants (including polychlorinated biphenyls, or PCBs) than wild salmon. And say no to sushi—raw fish often contains all sorts of parasites, from tapeworm larvae to liver flukes.

DON'T EAT: PROCESSED OR GENETICALLY MODIFIED OILS

Seeds are the most powerful sources of parent essential oils. The outer husk of the seed protects it from oxygen, which would oxidize the oil and destroy its ability to germinate. Oxidized oils are equally damaging to our body. When certain fragile oils are heated, they turn toxic and inflammatory, which is why PEOs must be organic, cold pressed, and minimally processed. (For info on the best oils for cooking, see pages 143–144.) The more polyunsaturated, the more fragile the oil. Proper oil extraction is performed by only a few small manufacturers, using cold-pressing techniques under a blanket of nitrogen to protect the oils from oxidative damage. Additionally, they should be packaged in dark or opaque bottles to shield them from light, which is one thousand times more deleterious to those delicate oils than is oxygen. They should be kept refrigerated.

Of course, this is not how most oil manufacturers do it! The vast majority use high pressures and temperatures to squeeze out the oils for mass production (corn, rapeseed, soy, sunflower, safflower, cottonseed, walnut, etc.), *which also squeezes out their nutritional value.* Sunflower, safflower, and soybean oils were once high in linoleic acid but are now high in oleic acid. Regardless of the quality of the seeds of origin, a heated MUFA or PUFA oil is nothing but toxic.

Stay away from non-organic and/or genetically modified oils, as they are typically contaminated with fat-soluble pesticides and other cell-damaging agents. Avoid genetically modified oils even if advertised as "cold processed."

DON'T EAT: CANOLA OIL (VEGETABLE OIL), PEANUT OIL, AND OTHER VERY-LONG-CHAIN FATTY ACIDS

When it comes to fatty acid molecules, size matters! Carbon chains of twenty-two or more present a problem because they're too long to be metabolized in your mitochondria, so they end up "dangling" outside mitochondrial membranes. This category includes canola oil (vegetable oil), peanut oil (and whole peanuts and peanut butter), and mustard oil. Although borage oil is rich in GLA, it is also one of the very-long-chain fatty acids so is best avoided.

DON'T EAT: TRANS FATS

I'm sure this isn't the first time you've heard this warning. Trans fats (a.k.a. hydrogenated fats or trans-fatty acids) are those with an altered molecular structure making them indigestible and toxic to your cells. Studies are clear that trans fats drive up inflammation, raise your risk for heart disease, and probably increase your risk for type 2 diabetes. The most common culprits are the partially hydrogenated vegetable oils found in margarine and butter substitutes.

The bottom line is, if you want to rev up your metabolism, you must feed your cells and heal their membranes because they oversee all metabolic operations. To keep them working like well-oiled machines, you need the right fats! Your diet should include a substantial intake of PEOs in that optimal 4:1 ratio.[27] These are precisely the foods featured in the Radical Metabolism plan!

To summarize what you've learned in this chapter, the following is a chart listing good fats and bad fats. For more information (including options for commercially prepared PEO products with omega oils already in the optimal ratio), refer to the fats section in Chapter 9.

FATS TO USE, FATS TO LOSE

FATS TO USE FRESH, ORGANIC, NON-GMO, COLD-PRESSED	FATS TO LOSE OXIDIZED, OVERHEATED, RANCID
Seeds and cold-pressed seed oils Hemp seed, hemp hearts, hemp oil High-linoleic safflower oil	Heated, processed, pressurized, and/or oxidized oils
Raw sunflower seeds, high-linoleic sunflower oil Rapeseed oil Sesame seeds and sesame oil	Non-organic and GMO oils
Flaxseed and high-lignan flaxseed oil Chia seed Pumpkin seeds and pumpkin seed oil Seed creams (soak overnight and blend)	Very-long-chain fatty acids (VLCFA): peanuts and peanut oil, canola oil (vegetable oil), mustard oil, borage oil
Black cumin seeds, a.k.a. black seed, black seed oil, black oil, black coriander oil Sacha inchi seeds, a.k.a. Incan peanuts Apricot seeds/kernels and apricot seed oil Clary sage seed oil	Trans-fatty acids
Raw nuts, nut oils, nut butters	Heated/roasted/irradiated nuts and nut products
Extra-virgin Siberian pine nut oil	
Avocados and avocado oil	
Whole olives and olive oil	
Spirulina	
Coconut, coconut oil, coconut cream, coconut milk, coconut yogurt, coconut manna (coconut butter)	
MCT oil	
Algae Oil	
Wild cold-water fish Salmon (low-mercury) Sardines Anchovies Caviar Tuna (low-mercury)	Farmed fish, sushi, and sashimi
Grass-pastured meat, poultry, eggs, and dairy (the last if you are not casein or lactose sensitive) Poultry Beef Lamb Buffalo Animal fats, such as tallow (beef dripping) and lard Cottage or ricotta cheese Hard cheese Cream Kefir Yogurt Butter Ghee	Conventionally raised meat, poultry, eggs, and dairy

3 RADICAL RULE #2: RESTORE YOUR GALLBLADDER

The voyage of discovery consists not in seeking new landscapes, but in having new eyes.

—Marcel Proust

IN THIS CHAPTER, YOU'LL LEARN . . .

- How bile is the forgotten switch for weight gain, hormone havoc, digestive problems, and body toxicity
- How sluggish bile may be derailing your thyroid
- The radical importance of your gallbladder, no matter what your doctor says
- How to know if your bile is toxic and congested
- The best fixes for building healthy bile—even if you no longer have your gallbladder
- How bitter foods jump-start slimming and improve your overall health

If you have been on other high-fat diets (think Paleo, Paleo Plus, Ketogenic, GAPS, or FODMAPS) and are still overweight, your gallbladder or lack thereof may be the reason why. And if your thyroid is slowing down, then—amazingly—your gallbladder may be the culprit here, too.

If you're like most people, you don't spend much time thinking about your gallbladder or how it relates to your metabolic situation. We go along in our busy lives blissfully unaware of the hard work this organ is doing on our behalf . . . all day, every day. Many experts talk about the importance of the liver and write volumes about toxicity without giving the gallbladder—or bile—so much as a passing nod.

Bile is the forgotten switch. Bile, although not the sexiest of topics, has several essential functions: It's what helps your body break down all those fats you eat, which are so critical for healthy cell membranes. And bile carries away all the toxins and hormone metabolites from your body. You see, not only is bile the real key to your ability to digest and assimilate fats, but it is also a vehicle for removing toxins so they can be flushed out of your liver. Bile is one of your body's premier (albeit underrated) detox mechanisms. Therefore, the consequences of toxic bile go far beyond the inability to lose weight. If your liver can't clean fats, then it most likely cannot break down hormones or other metabolic waste products, either.

In this chapter, we will connect the dots between the gallbladder and liver, bile, metabolism, weight gain, and hormone dysfunction. In fact, the bile connection may very well be your first clue to a sluggish thyroid, as you will later discover!

Gallbladder disease and obesity are both occurring at epidemic rates. Problems with fat digestion have come into focus with today's higher-fat diets, such as Paleo and Ketogenic types. We are finally breaking up with sugar and starting a new love affair with fats—*and this is a good thing*. But for many this new romance has gotten off to a rocky start. Some of the folks who have trouble digesting fats simply quit these diets when they feel worse instead of better, not realizing that the real problem isn't the higher-fat diet, but instead compromised gallbladder function and sluggish bile. Bile is the missing link—you simply can't be healthy without it.

IS YOUR METABOLISM STUCK DUE TO TOXIC, SLUGGISH BILE?

Here's a little biochemistry 101 for you. Together, your liver and gallbladder make up your hepatic system. When your hepatic system is functioning well, you'll have good circulation, clean blood, and a healthy cellular metabolism.

The liver is so essential that you could only survive for a day or two if it stopped functioning altogether. It is one of the largest organs in the body, weighing in at around 3 pounds/1.3kg, and is situated on the right side of your upper abdomen, just below your diaphragm. As the body's prime detoxification organ, the liver takes an enormous beating from today's toxic world. Many foods and lifestyle factors, such as refined sugar and grains, unhealthy fats, too little fiber, too much alcohol and caffeine, medications, and emotional stress, are quite hard on the liver.

Your liver is the only organ that can rebuild itself—up to 75 percent of it can be damaged and it can still regenerate if given the proper nutritional support. The most prevalent liver disease today is non-alcoholic fatty liver disease (NAFLD), which is characterized by the accumulation of fat in the liver. This is really a sign that the liver has stopped processing fat and begun storing it. NAFLD rates have doubled since 1988 and are linked to obesity, diabetes, hypertension, and lipid imbalances. NAFLD often goes undetected and can progress into something even more serious, for which the end result can be complete liver failure.

If your liver is sluggish, every organ in your body is affected and your weight-loss efforts will be stalled from multiple angles. *A fatty liver is a toxic liver,* as one of its responsibilities is to neutralize the myriad of toxins that assault our bodies every day. If you have a roll of belly fat, you may have a fatty liver. When your liver becomes clogged up with pollutants and metabolic waste, not only does fat accumulate in and around it, but also around your other organs and throughout the body. Cellulite, weight gain, and increased visceral fat are all signs your liver may be suffering from toxic overload, and this is really a downer for your metabolism. You will lose excess body fat only when your hepatic function is restored.

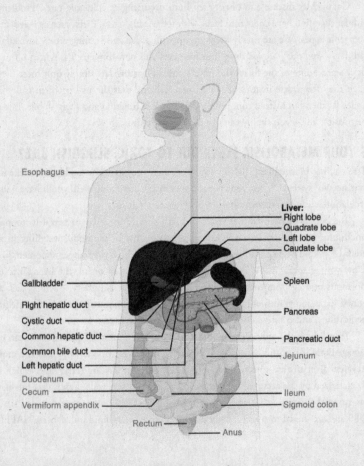

The same factors that have so stressed our livers have dealt equally devastating blows to our gallbladders and bile flow—and yet no one is giving you this important information.

THE GALLBLADDER AND BILE

Believe it or not, bile plays a pivotal role in your body's ability to remain slim and trim. But first, you have to understand a little basic anatomy and physiology. Your gallbladder is your liver's best friend and vital to its operations. The liver secretes about a litre and a half of bile daily (also called gall), storing and concentrating it in your gallbladder. Bile breaks down dietary fats into smaller particles that are more digestible and absorbable. When you eat fats, bile is released from your gallbladder into your intestine via the bile duct.

Adequate, healthy bile is essential for your body to absorb those all-important fatty acids you learned about in Chapter 2. It also helps you absorb fat-soluble vitamins, such as vitamin A (the infection fighter), vitamin E (the fertility vitamin), vitamin K (the bone healer), and vitamin D (the healing, hormone-like vitamin that boosts immunity and wards off breast and colon cancers). Fats are precursors to every hormone, so not digesting them has major consequences. If undigested fat globules pass from your gut into your bloodstream, then your cells cannot incorporate them into cell membranes, and your body has no choice other than to store them on your derriere.

Decades of consuming processed foods and nutritionally impoverished low-fat and non-fat diets, compounded by unending toxic exposures, have quietly damaged our gallbladder function, leading to thick, overconcentrated, and congested bile—which I call toxic bile. Toxic bile is thick, sticky bile that has stopped flowing freely, so it's no longer able to perform its duties. Bile can turn toxic from excess cholesterol, high toxin load, clogged bile ducts, or insufficient intake of the specific nutrients that keep it thin and flowing. Studies also link elevated blood sugar levels to thicker bile and gallstone formation.

Toxic bile and obesity feed off each other. In an animal study, obese subjects secreted and released only half as much bile as did their leaner counterparts.[1] One 2016 study published in the American Heart Association's journal *Arteriosclerosis, Thrombosis, and Vascular Biology* showed that gallstones come with a 23 percent increased risk of coronary artery disease.[2] When your bile is sick, you get sick—it's that simple.

In addition to fat digestion, bile plays a major role in detoxification—flushing out all the toxins your liver collects. Like a magnet, bile grabs onto all sorts of nasty stuff so it can be eliminated from your body in the feces. Bile is an unseemly brew of such things as heavy metals, drugs, foreign chemicals, food preservatives, contaminants (e.g. pesticides and flame retardants)—whatever the liver is getting rid of goes into the bile.

The problem is, if your bile is thick and congested and not flowing, all that sludge sticks around in your body. Those excess toxins get stored in your fat cells. Think about it—*your body has to put them somewhere!* This promotes cellulite by increasing deposition of body fat and reducing collagen formation.

As toxins accumulate, your health declines. Toxic overload is a big factor in much of the chronic disease we see today. The quantity and quality of your bile is directly proportional to the number of toxins it can eliminate. By the time people develop allergies, arthritis, and joint inflammation, they have a 75 percent bile deficiency, and by the time they develop a major chronic illness, such as cancer or heart disease, their bile production is compromised by a whopping 90 percent. Toxic bile is associated with numerous health problems, including obesity, hormone imbalance, hypothyroidism, autoimmune issues, and more.

GALLSTONES

If you begin experiencing nausea, vomiting, pain, fatigue, or a mélange of other problems, it could be your gallbladder sending out a major SOS.

When bile becomes sludgy, gallstones begin to form. Gallstones are hard masses that develop in the gallbladder or bile ducts. They are composed of cholesterol and calcium bilirubinate or calcium carbonate and can get quite large—up to the size of a golf ball.[3] Most people with gallstones experience no overt symptoms because the stones accumulate in the gallbladder and don't move beyond there, but sometimes the gallbladder becomes inflamed (cholecystitis). Unresolved symptoms you may never have connected to your gallbladder or bile may include

- Hypothyroidism (sign of deficient bile to stimulate active thyroid hormone in fat cells)
- Constipation (inadequate bile for lubrication)
- Nausea or vomiting (not enough bile)
- Pain that comes on suddenly and quickly worsens; pain is generally focused on the right side, just below the rib cage, between the shoulder blades, in the right shoulder, or up the right side of the neck
- Headache over the eyes
- Burping, gas, bloating, constant feeling of fullness
- Gastroesophageal reflux (GERD)
- Bitter taste in the mouth after meals (bile reflux)
- Light-colored or floating stools (lack of bile output)
- Hemorrhoids (congested liver)
- Inability to lose weight

- Fibromyalgia (liver and gallbladder toxicity)
- Mood changes such as irritability, depression, or anxiety
- Dry skin and hair (essential fatty acid deficiency)
- Varicose veins
- History of prescription or recreational drug use (need for more liver and gallbladder support)
- Easily intoxicated (need for more liver and gallbladder support)

If gallstones go on the move, they sometimes get stuck in the gallbladder opening or in the bile duct, and cause severe upper abdominal pain in the center, or just right of center. Typically, the pain begins within an hour of eating, especially after a high-fat meal, and lasts a few hours before subsiding although it may continue longer in waves. If an obstruction is severe enough, it can cause a life-threatening gallbladder infection. This type of infection most often ends with hospitalization and gallbladder surgery. Pancreatitis is another complication when a gallstone passes through the bile duct and blocks the pancreatic duct. If bile seeps into the bloodstream, signs of jaundice (yellowing of the skin and whites of the eyes) may appear. Unfortunately, many people are unaware they have a gallbladder problem or gallstones until they experience a medical crisis, making prevention paramount.

Gallbladder removal is the most frequently performed abdominal surgery in the United States today.[4] Unlike your liver, your gallbladder cannot regenerate itself. Those who lose their gallbladder experience increased risk for obesity, in addition to a number of serious health problems.[5]

> Myth: You don't really need your gallbladder.

Contrary to the fact that many physicians still tell their patients that losing their gallbladder is no big deal, not having one puts you at a serious disadvantage. Bile is not vile—*bile is brilliant!* Think of your gallbladder as the tank and bile as the oil. Your gallbladder was concentrating the bile it received from your liver and mixing it with salts and enzymes. Without the holding tank, bile has nowhere to go except straight into your small intestine in a continuous trickle, regardless of the presence or absence of dietary fat. The failure to match bile output with fat consumption compromises your ability to properly digest the fats you eat, resulting in nutritional deficiencies—and expanding waistlines.

It is very common to experience weight gain after gallbladder removal. Animal studies tell us that triglyceride levels increase in both the blood and liver, as does VLDL production. VLDL stands for "very low-density lipoproteins," which are the most dangerous kind of LDL. Recirculation of bile acids also increases, which affects energy balance, body weight, glucose levels, insulin sensitivity, and cholesterol regulation. Research suggests the risk of metabolic syndrome, type 2 diabetes, heart disease, and fatty liver all rise substantially after gallbladder surgery.[6]

Even if you still have your gallbladder, if your bile is not flowing properly, you may experience many of the same problems as people who have had their gallbladder removed. Whether or not you still have your gallbladder, there are steps you can take to support your bile.

BILE ACIDS AND BILE SALTS? THINK: DETERGENT

Don't let bile terminology bog you down! Bile is basically a degreasing agent—*like detergent.* Thanks to bile acids and bile salts (which are essentially different forms of the same thing), bile is able to break down larger fat globules into smaller fat droplets (emulsification), so that your enzymes (lipases) can fully digest them.

Bile acids are made from cholesterol and represent about 80 percent of the organic compounds in bile. After their synthesis by the liver, they are combined with the amino acids taurine and glycine to form primary bile acids, which make them water-soluble and better able to emulsify fats. These combined forms are known as bile salts. In the small intestine, bile salts are converted by bacteria into secondary bile acids.

As large quantities of bile acids are flushed into your small intestine every day, 95 percent are absorbed back into your blood and returned to your liver. The remaining 5 percent are excreted in the stool. In your colon, bile acids draw in water and increase motility, preventing constipation. If bile acids are not properly reabsorbed from the colon, a condition called bile acid diarrhea can develop, characterized by chronic bloating, urgency, and watery diarrhea. Bile acid diarrhea is often misdiagnosed as irritable bowel syndrome (IBS) and is estimated to affect about 1 percent of the population.[7]

Bile acids are also closely tied to blood sugar and are typically deficient in individuals with type 2 diabetes or insulin resistance. Many studies show that proper bile release is important for balancing blood sugar.[8]

Because bile salts are derived from cholesterol, bile is also instrumental in regulating cholesterol levels in your body. Approximately 80 percent of your body's cholesterol is used by the liver to produce bile salts—roughly 500 milligrams every day. Since bile salts are a primary component of bile, adding more into the diet helps the liver to make more bile. This is especially helpful after gallbladder surgery.

THE #1 NUTRIENT FOR BETTER BILE

Let's think back to those cell membranes. As you learned in Chapter 1, cell membranes are made of fats: phospholipids and cholesterol. Guess what? These same phospholipids are also a critical component of bile.

Choline is a very important nutrient in every cell in your body, first discovered in bile. The choline in bile helps with emulsification of fats, making them water-soluble. Choline is involved in tons of other processes as well, such as lipid transport, liver repair, nerve conductivity, brain development, and cognition.[9] Choline helps control the deposition of fat in your organs, especially in the liver—so significantly that choline deficiency can directly cause fatty liver disease.[10] Choline also helps keep homocysteine levels low, which is important because high levels of homocysteine raise your cardiovascular risk.

Choline deficiency is a deal-breaker for bile production and also leads to muscle damage. Up to 90 percent of women over age forty are choline deficient.

You can obtain choline from food sources, such as beef, almonds, cauliflower, haricot beans, and amaranth. Although eggs are also a rich source of choline, I recommend avoiding them because they are the most highly allergic food for the gallbladder (see page 49). The recommended daily allowance for choline is 425 milligrams for women and 550 for men, but I recommend 500 mg *with each meal* for both men and women, which is nearly triple the RDA—at least for a few weeks. After that, you can decrease the dose to once or twice a day (with meals). This amount is particularly helpful for those with fatty liver disease.

Lecithin contains choline in varying amounts, and has been shown to support bile flow, cholesterol balance and optimal lipid profiles, cell membranes, and overall brain and nervous system function.[11] My experience with patients, as well as myself, has been that lecithin supplements have offered some benefits, such as accelerating fat loss, improving digestion, and relieving constipation, gas, and bloating. However, newer studies have uncovered some concerns, so I am no longer recommending lecithin supplements. Of particular concern is a recent study suggesting lecithin is metabolized by some people's gut flora into a metabolite that shows up in high concentrations in those who suffer heart attack or stroke, a compound called trimethylamine N-oxide (TMAO).[12] This is a correlation—not a causation—so we still don't know whether this compound plays a causative role in those events. Nevertheless, it is enough for me to withdraw my recommendations about lecithin as there are safer options available for getting your choline.

CONDITIONS STEMMING FROM TOXIC BILE

No matter how balanced your diet, without healthy bile you simply can't get those fabulous fat-blasting, membrane-protecting, fuel-providing benefits. But beyond your

Toxic Bile

GERD

IBD

Parasites

Food Allergies

Constipation

Weight gain

Leaky Gut

Nausea

Yeast

Type 2 Diabetes

Thyroid Issues

Autoimmunity

Indigestion

Depression

Cellulite

Hormone Imbalance

metabolism, toxic bile and gallbladder dysfunction are now linked to a shocking laundry list of other diseases, including GERD, thyroid issues, autoimmune problems, hormone dysregulation—and the list goes on. This is quite concerning because the majority of individuals with bile and gallbladder disease are completely unaware they *have* a bile or gallbladder problem.

When it comes to people seeking help for digestive ailments, the last decade has brought hundreds if not thousands of books about leaky gut syndrome, small intestine bacterial overgrowth (SIBO), IBS, detox and cleansing, inflammation, autoimmunity, thyroid dysfunction, and the like—yet no one has addressed the importance of bile. Between 1 and 1.3 million Americans suffer from inflammatory bowel disease (IBD)[13] and up to 80 percent of those also have SIBO.[14] Leaky gut is occurring in epidemic numbers. Bile is a factor in *all* these conditions—if your gut is not healthy, no amount of intervention will fix the problem unless you also address the bile. I believe this is one of the major reasons so many people are sick today. The problem is even worse if you've had your gallbladder removed.

When you try to treat a condition without knowing the underlying cause, you get treatments that don't work but are just palliative measures that temporarily reduce symptoms without correcting the underlying problem. With this approach, symptoms tend to recur and even worsen because the causative factor has been ignored. Greater and greater stress is placed on your immune system.

Let's take a closer look at a few more common conditions associated with toxic bile.

WHEN CONSTIPATION COMES TO CALL

Believe it or not, constipation is a common symptom of toxic bile, and for good reason. Bile salts are responsible for lubricating the intestinal tract, so if you have bile insufficiency, constipation is the natural consequence. As you increase your bile flow, constipation may become no more than an unpleasant memory. Simply implementing the dietary strategies to incorporate bitter foods that you'll find later in this chapter will go a long way toward eliminating constipation.

Be sure to move your body and drink plenty of water every day. Exercise gets everything moving—blood, lymph, bile, and bowels. One study found that exercise reduced the risk of gallstones by one third.[15] Something as simple as drinking a large glass of water first thing in the morning may help prevent gallstones. Drinking water has been shown to induce gallbladder contractions, therefore causing the gallbladder to empty. Other beverages may have a similar effect. Chewing food slowly also gives the body time to produce more bile.

HEARTBURN AND ACID REFLUX

Do you experience acid reflux, heartburn, or GERD? Have you been told your symptoms are from overproduction of stomach acid? This brings us to another myth!

Myth: GERD is caused by excess stomach acid.

Almost everyone has been brainwashed into believing excess stomach acid is the root of their digestive issues, yet there is no evidence for this. In fact, studies show the opposite—GERD is more often associated with *underproduction* of stomach acid (hydrochloric acid, or HCl). GERD, commonly called acid indigestion, occurs when your stomach contents backflush into the esophagus and cause a burning sensation, or heartburn. GERD can also produce gas, bloating, or burping shortly after a meal. Individuals typically experience a 40 percent drop in stomach acid production by the time they reach their thirties, and another 50 percent decrease by age seventy. In one study, almost one third of individuals over age sixty produced little to no stomach acid.[16] Over time, reflux can have some serious complications, such as esophageal inflammation, erosion, ulceration, bleeding, scarring, and even esophageal cancer, so you do not want to let this continue.

If heartburn is not caused by excess stomach acid, then what *is* the cause? GERD is almost always a muscle problem, specifically of the valve at the lower end of the esophagus called the lower esophageal sphincter (LES). This valve is supposed to keep gastric juices from backing up into your esophagus, except when you belch or vomit. However, in people with GERD, the LES fails to close properly, allowing stomach contents to pass through. Reflux produces symptoms regardless of how much or how little acid is in your stomach—*the problem is not excess acid, but rather acid in the wrong place*. Why does the LES malfunction? One reason is increased stomach pressure, such as from overeating. Another is gas related to poor digestion of certain carbohydrates or sugars that ferment in the stomach. Dairy is a major offender, due to lactose. Other foods can weaken the LES, such as alcoholic beverages, acidic foods, spicy foods, coffee, and chocolate, as well as certain medications.

The conventional treatment for GERD is to block normal stomach acid production, using antacids (Tums, Rennie), H2 blockers (Zantac, Tagamet), and proton-pump inhibitors (PPIs; these include Prilosec, Prevacid, and Nexium). Millions of people have been popping PPIs on a daily basis to suppress their acid production—*and the majority had a low-acid problem to begin with.* Therefore, it's no surprise these drugs have created a boatload of side effects, ranging from digestive problems and nutritional deficiencies to impaired immunity.

You might be wondering what GERD and stomach acid have to do with your gallbladder. Well, low HCl and gallbladder problems go hand in hand. When you eat, hydrochloric acid is what triggers the release of bile (via the hormone cholecystokinin) as well as the release of pancreatic enzymes—so blocking HCl stops bile flow. Excess dietary carbohydrates and starches, as well as insufficient fats, can stifle HCl and impair bile production. Stress, overeating, eating too quickly, eating irregularly, not chewing your food thoroughly, and drinking large amounts of fluids with meals can all challenge your body's HCl production. Making matters worse, popping PPIs at the first sign of heartburn only further impairs the bile, so you're trading temporary relief for a far more serious problem that may eventually cost you your gallbladder—or worse.

Before looking at how you can increase stomach acid production, there is one more issue worth mentioning. The pylorus, also known as the pyloric valve—the valve between your stomach and small intestine—should be like a one-way door from your stomach into your intestine, but it can become spastic. A spastic pylorus can cause bile to flow backward, from your small intestine into your stomach (bile reflux), and this produces symptoms similar to acid reflux, such as bloating, pain, nausea, and vomiting.

Hydrochloric acid has many beneficial functions for your health. Besides triggering bile release, HCl also reduces gas by helping break down carbohydrates before they can be fermented and kills gas-producing bacteria in your small intestine. It also plays an important role in protein digestion, which we'll address in the next chapter. By making your stomach highly acidic, HCl also protects you from pathogenic bacteria and parasites that may have hitched a ride with your brunch.

How do you boost your hydrochloric acid levels? Many find relief taking a stomach acid replacement, such as apple cider vinegar before meals. However, if your esophageal lining is damaged or you have a hiatal hernia, you may not be able to tolerate more acid until those tissues are healed. The best solution is to correct the condition

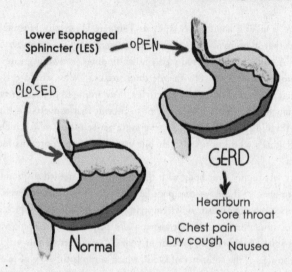

that's blocking normal acid production in the first place, instead of artificially raising it. Some of the causes have already been discussed, but also make sure you are getting plenty of HCl-supporting nutrients, such as sodium, iodine, and zinc—think: seafood and pumpkin seeds. Don't overdo protein, as this can overwhelm HCl production. Make sure you're getting plenty of vitamin C because low vitamin C will suppress conversion of cholesterol into bile.[17] Other helpful treatments include papaya leaf, bromelain, and pine nut oil. For more about GERD and HCl, I highly recommend Dr. Jonathon Wright's book *Why Stomach Acid Is Good for You.*[18]

WITHOUT GOOD BILE, YOUR THYROID MAY CRASH

Few people realize that sluggish bile can actually drag down your thyroid. *If you're not absorbing fats, you can't make thyroid hormone. Period.*

Around 80 percent of women over the age of forty suffer from insufficient, poor-quality bile, and suboptimal bile flow and sluggish thyroid share many of the same symptoms, including fatigue, weight gain, digestive issues, constipation, leptin resistance, dry skin, and many more. According to the American Thyroid Association, more than 12 percent of Americans will develop a thyroid condition during their lifetime. Twenty million Americans have some form of thyroid disease, but up to 60 percent of them are unaware of their condition.[19] Evidence is mounting that hypothyroidism is linked to congested bile.

Scientists from Harvard and others overseas have discovered the missing link between thyroid and bile in several landmark studies—but the shocking truth is that no one is talking about it. A study at Tampere University Hospital in Finland found that hypothyroidism is *seven times more likely in people with reduced bile flow*.[20] A study at Tufts produced similar findings, showing greater rates of hypothyroidism among those with bile duct stones.[21] Why would this be? The reason is that bile acids boost thyroid activity.[22] According to thyroid specialist Dr. Antonio Bianco, bile triggers the release of an enzyme that converts T4 (the body's less active thyroid hormone) into T3 (the more active form), which fuels metabolism. Individuals who improved their bile experienced an enormous increase in metabolism.[23]

Dietary fats supply your body with the raw materials needed to produce active thyroid hormones, so it follows that poor fat digestion lowers thyroid levels. Making matters worse, hypothyroidism slows emptying of the biliary tract, which increases your risk for stone formation.[24] Gut bacteria also play a role in helping your body convert T4 into T3—about 20 percent of your T4 is converted this way. Thyroid hormone also relaxes the sphincter of Oddi, which controls the flow of bile into the small intestine. If your thyroid hormone levels are low, this sphincter tenses up and less bile can pass, which increases the risk for gallstones.[25] Even now with all this groundbreaking science, more than 90 percent of physicians fail to recognize bile as a factor for their thyroid patients.

AUTOIMMUNE CONDITIONS

Rates of autoimmune disease have tripled over the last few decades, and it's no accident that autoimmune disorders can be associated with a 75 percent drop in bile production. Estimates are that between 24 and 50 million Americans now suffer from autoimmune conditions—typically more than one.[26] Autoimmunity affects more women than heart disease and breast cancer combined and is one of the top ten causes of death for girls and women in all age groups, up to sixty-four.[27] One of the main causes is toxicity, and as you know bile is integral to detoxification. (We will be talking more about toxicity in Chapter 6.)

Of special concern is Hashimoto's thyroiditis (HT), which by some estimates accounts for 90 to 95 percent of hypothyroidism cases.[28] HT is the most prevalent autoimmune disorder and occurs when the immune system attacks thyroid tissue. *Even the most astute Hashimoto's researchers are missing the bile connection.* The prevalence of HT is reported to be about 5 percent of the population,[29] but this estimate is actually quite low because so many are asymptomatic in its early stages. HT is five to ten times more common in women than men, and its prevalence is on the rise.[30] Forty-three percent of those with Hashimoto's are estimated to have gluten sensitivity, which we will be discussing in Chapter 5.[31]

There have been many helpful natural supplements for those with Hashimoto's, ranging from thiamine to HCL and selenium. But one recent discovery that shows promise for those with Hashimoto's thyroiditis is black seed (*Nigella sativa*). One study showed the condition can be improved by simply adding 2 grams of powdered black seed to your daily diet.[32] Black seed is a rich source of those parent omega-6 EFAs that strengthen cell membranes and improve cellular communication—*and autoimmune diseases are all about cellular communication*. The body is not communicating well with itself.

FOOD ALLERGIES AND SENSITIVITIES

You have probably not heard food allergies and the gallbladder mentioned in the same sentence, but according to the late Dr. James C. Brenemen, former chairman of the Food Allergy Committee of the American College of Allergists, there is a significant correlation between gallbladder dysfunction and food allergies. Dr. Brenemen tracked allergies among gallbladder patients and identified the three top offenders: eggs (93 percent of individuals), pork (64 percent), and onions (52 percent).[33] When you have a sensitivity to these foods, consuming them produces edema in the bile ducts, which interferes with bile release. The good news is that removing the offending foods from the diet *for as little as one week* can bring relief from gallbladder pain and possibly prevent gallbladder surgery down the road.

TOXIC BILE, ESTROGEN DOMINANCE, AND "FALSE FAT"

Is perimenopause or menopause hitting you like a runaway train? Are you lying awake night after night with hot flashes, insomnia, and brain fog? In my opinion, hormone imbalance among women is twice as common today as one hundred years ago. One of the ways to restore hormone balance is to build healthy bile. Bile is your ticket to detox. *Toxic, sluggish bile, and hormone problems go hand in hand.*

My hunch is that 80 percent of women over age forty have bile insufficiency. Women have an increased risk of bile problems and gallstones because estrogen stimulates the liver to remove more cholesterol from the blood and divert it into the bile, causing bile to thicken. Elevated blood sugars further complicate the problem. It's no surprise that 25 percent of American women have gallstones by the age of sixty, and 50 percent have them by age seventy-five.[34] And it's a vicious (and viscous) cycle—once your bile has thickened, it's less able to break down excess estrogen.

Most women are too high in estrogen producing a condition called estrogen dominance. Estrogen is present in everything from oral contraceptives to hormone replacement therapy (HRT) to xenoestrogens (synthetic estrogen-mimicking compounds in pesticides and food additives). Estrogen dominance leads to a wide range of issues, including decreased sex drive, irregular periods, PMS, breast tenderness or fibrocystic breasts, headaches, mood swings, fatigue, hypothyroidism, hair loss, foggy thinking—and more serious problems, such as autoimmunity, breast cancer, and infertility. Estrogen is necessary for serotonin production by affecting how the body metabolizes tryptophan, serotonin's precursor. Serotonin deficiency can lead to food cravings, weight gain, and depression.

In addition to contributing to body fat, estrogen dominance is notorious for causing something I refer to as "false fat." False fat is fluid trapped in body tissues that contributes to bloating, puffiness, and cellulite. Many of us women carry an extra 10 to 15 pounds/4 to 6kg of it. Some of us—15 to 25 percent—are more salt sensitive than others, so be careful about the amount as well as the type of salt you consume. Choose natural sea salt as opposed to common table salt, as sea salt is lower in sodium and provides valuable trace minerals. Include more fresh vegetables and fruits in your diet, which tend to be rich in potassium. Potassium is an important mineral that helps balance out sodium in the body. Restaurant food is typically very high in sodium, so you might want to make better use of your own kitchen. In addition to high sodium and estrogen levels, fluid retention may also come from food sensitivities (see Chapter 5), adrenal stress, or dysregulated insulin.

HOW TO DIAGNOSE A GALLBLADDER PROBLEM

Do you think your gallbladder might be unhealthy? Are your symptoms suspicious but you want confirmation? There are some tests that can be helpful but you'll have to be proactive. I'm sorry to say, your health-care practitioner may not have you covered in this area—*less than 10 percent of physicians think to test for bile flow*.

BLOOD TESTS

Signs of a gallbladder problem can sometimes be picked up first on routine blood panels, so consider including a few basic blood tests in your routine preventative care. You can't assume your gallbladder is healthy just because you're *not* having symptoms. If you suspect a gallbladder problem, a variety of tests can be helpful or confirmatory. For example, sometimes an infection is identified in a complete blood count (CBC) if white blood cells are elevated. Other tests can reveal high bilirubin levels, which indicate jaundice, a complication of gallbladder problems. Liver function tests look for elevated enzymes that may reveal a biliary obstruction.

There are three primary liver enzymes that can be measured in the blood: ALT (alanine aminotransferase), AST (aspartate aminotransferase), and GGT (gamma-glutamyl transferase). All three are found predominantly in the liver but to a lesser extent in other organs (muscles, heart, kidneys, pancreas, spleen, brain, testes, etc.). Normally these enzyme levels are low, but when your liver is diseased or damaged, they are released into your bloodstream and cause levels to rise. Diagnostics are tricky, therefore liver function tests are only helpful when considered as part of the overall picture.

In healthy individuals, ALT and AST levels can vary from 10 to 45 percent in a single day, as well as differing by race and ethnicity. Your highest ALT levels typically occur in the afternoon and the lowest at night. Besides biliary obstruction, elevated ALT and AST can be caused by many things, such as cirrhosis, heart attack, strenuous exercise, certain viral infections, tobacco, alcohol, and certain medications. Moderate exercise can increase AST to almost three times the normal limit for up to 24 hours. If only AST is elevated, it relates to the heart, but if both AST and GGT are up, then it could be your gallbladder.

Your GGT level is not a standard test—you'll probably have to request it. GGT among African Americans tends to be twice as high as Caucasians, and 25 to 50 percent higher in obese individuals. Low GGT may indicate hypothyroidism or magnesium deficiency. All these variables can make liver enzyme interpretation somewhat challenging, so you'll need an astute health-care practitioner to help you sort it all out.

DIAGNOSTIC IMAGING TESTS

Your physician may need to see a visual of your liver and gallbladder to make a diagnosis. Imaging procedures all have their strengths and weaknesses. Abdominal X-rays can spot some calcium-containing gallstones, but not all types. Computed tomography (CT) scans are not the best way to look for gallstones but can detect a rupture or infection in the gallbladder or bile ducts. Ultrasound is the most commonly used imaging test for detecting all sizes of gallstones, but it tells you nothing about inflammation. Magnetic resonance imaging (MRI) is sometimes helpful for seeing stones in the bile ducts but can miss tiny stones or infections. There are other tests as well, but these are the most commonly used.

RESTORE YOUR GALLBLADDER— AND GIVE GALLSTONES THE BOOT

Now that you understand the importance of bile and why your gallbladder is anything but a throwaway organ, let's turn our focus to what you can do to improve bile production and gallbladder tone. This is a substantial part of creating a radical metabolism, and as usual diet is key. If you have symptoms of impaired fat digestion, such as nausea, bloating, constipation, or pale stools, or if you've had your gallbladder removed, then it's wise—I might even say critical—to increase your intake of bile-building foods and consider supplements to improve bile flow. Laying some love on your liver and gallbladder will add years to your life and life to your years. There are simple, effective strategies, even if you've had your gallbladder removed.

If you are living with an intermittently unhappy gallbladder, please be familiar with the danger signs that indicate a need for immediate medical attention:

- Upper-right quadrant pain that does not go away within 5 hours
- Fever or vomiting
- Changes in bowel movement and urine

If you have the above, then you should get evaluated ASAP. Chances are, however, that if you're reading this book your symptoms are less severe and more chronic in nature. There are a number of natural treatments you can do at home to reduce inflammation and restore healthy bile flow, whether you have a gallbladder or not. If you could do *only one thing* to improve the situation, it would be to incorporate more bitter foods into your diet—so this is our first strategy.

THE BEAUTY OF BITTERS

Many plant foods qualify as bitters. Studies suggest bitters "get your juices flowing" (literally) by stimulating the release of bile, as well as saliva, HCl, pepsin, gastrin, and pancreatic enzymes. Bitters may also increase the tone of your lower esophageal sphincter (LES). It is unclear if we even need to swallow the bitters—some research suggests we only need to *taste them* for them to be effective, which makes bitters effective in relatively small doses.

A good starting point is to wean yourself off sweet tastes and develop a new love of bitter. We have lost our natural affinity for bitter foods and traded it in for a pervasive and ultimately dangerous sugar addiction. This addiction to sweets has sabotaged any semblance of a "balanced diet" and opened a Pandora's box of health problems. Americans are consuming between 35 and 70kg of sugar every year—and that's just table sugar and does not include other refined carbohydrates.[35] Years of processed food and low-fat diets, high in sugar and refined carbohydrates, have contributed to sluggish gallbladders and congested bile, among other things. We didn't have this problem when we were eating off the farm!

The antidote to "sweet addiction" is the development of other tastes. Your tongue has sensors for sweet, salty, sour, and bitter tastes—and the more you cut back on the sweet, the better you'll develop the other three. Bitter greens, such as watercress, rocket, endive (chicory), dandelion, and radicchio, offer wonderful benefits, as does horseradish, which also has cancer-fighting properties. The following table lists a wide variety of bitter foods to incorporate in your diet—and many may surprise you!

BITTER FOODS

BITTER FOODS: VEGETABLES & FRUITS

Alfalfa	Artichoke	Arugula (rocket)
Asparagus	Aubergine	Beet greens (beetroot tops)
Bitter gourd (bitter melon, karela)	Broccoli	Brussels sprouts
Cabbage	Cauliflower	Cucumbers
Daikon radish (mooli)	Dandelion greens	Endive (chicory, escarole)
Frisée	Grapefruit	Jerusalem artichokes
Jicama (yam bean)	Kale	Lemon and lemon rind
Lime and lime rind	Lotus leaf	Mizuna
Mustard greens	Nettles	Olives (uncured)
Orange peel	Puntarelle	Radicchio
Radish	Rapini (cime di rapa)	Red leaf lettuce
Rhubarb root	Romaine lettuce	Spinach
Spring greens	Swiss chard	Tatsoi
Thistles	Turnips and turnip greens	Watercress or cress
Wild lettuce	Winter purslane (miners' lettuce)	

BITTER FOODS: HERBS & SPICES

Angelica	Angostura bark	Anise
Barberry bark	Basil	Bergamot
Burdock root	Caraway	Cardamom
Chamomile	Chicory root	Cinnamon
Coriander	Dill	Fennel
Fenugreek seeds	Garlic	Gentian root
Ginger	Goldenseal root	Hops flowers
Horehound	Horseradish	Milk thistle
Mint	Parsley	Rue
Saffron	Scutellaria	Sorrel
Thyme	Turmeric	Wormwood leaf
Yarrow flower	Yellow dock	

BITTER FOODS: OTHER

Aloe vera	Apricot seeds and seed oil	Bitter orange
Bittersweet chocolate	Cacao	Coffee
Peach stones	Plum stones	Seaweed (dulse, arame, nori, kombu, wakame, etc.)
Sesame	Vinegar	

HERBAL BITTERS

Bitter foods as well as bitter herbs can significantly boost digestion, which is how digestive bitters came about, and today there are many formulas from which to choose. According to Dr. Wright in *Why Stomach Acid Is Good for You*, the most commonly used herbs in Western herbal medicine are the following:

- Barberry bark
- Caraway
- Dandelion
- Fennel
- Gentian root
- Ginger
- Globe artichoke
- Goldenseal root
- Hops flowers
- Milk thistle
- Peppermint
- Wormwood
- Yellow dock

Herbal bitters formulas are available in just about any natural food store and usually are tinctures of several bitter herbs. Digestive bitters are completely plant-based, therefore accessible if you're vegan or vegetarian. I suggest taking the recommended dose (typically 5 to 10 drops) in as little water as possible about 15 minutes before a meal, and after a meal as needed for heartburn, indigestion, or bloating. Be careful if you have severe GERD, and go lightly if your stomach lining is compromised. If you get nauseous, back off on the dose. You can even make your own digestive bitters. Mountain Rose Herbs offers a simple recipe calling for dandelion root, fennel seed, ginger, and orange peel.[36] Stay away from Swedish bitters, as they typically contain herbal laxatives, such as rhubarb and senna.

Ever heard of Angostura bitters? A very popular brand of cocktail bitters, these were named after a Venezuelan town formerly named Angostura, but now called Ciudad Bolivar. Legend has it that this secret formula contains an extract from the bark of the angostura plant, a shrublike citrus tree native to that region. A bitter chemical in the bark called angosturin is a quinolone that's regarded as a good digestive and antibacterial. (You might recognize another variety of quinolone found in tonic water and some types of vermouth: quinine, an antimalarial.) The principal ingredient in Angostura bitters is listed as gentian root, but the formula is a well-kept secret—whether or not it actually contains angostura bark extract is anyone's guess, but it makes for entertaining culinary lore.[37]

An alternative to digestive bitters is the juice of naturally fermented sauerkraut, which is acidic and loaded with gut-friendly microbes. Start with one teaspoon and work your way up two to three tablespoons before each meal. In Chapter 5 we will talk more about gut health and the microbiome.

BRILLIANT BILE-BUILDERS

In addition to bitter greens and such, other ingredients and supplements are especially good for bile and gallbladder support.

Look for a supplement that contains some or all of the "superstar six" for building bile: choline, taurine, beetroot, pancreatic lipase, ox bile, and collinsonia root.

Beetroots: Beetroots contain betaine, a rich source of HCl that thins the bile and helps prevent gallstones.

Choline: A major component of bile that helps emulsify fats; a vitamin-like nutrient present in every cell in your body. For more about choline, see page 43.

Taurine: A key component of bile acids, this essential amino acid helps bile excrete chemicals detoxed by the liver, increases bile acid production and thins the bile, and reduces cholesterol levels in the blood and liver. Many people are deficient, especially vegans and vegetarians, because taurine is derived from organ meats and other animal tissues. Taurine also improves lipid profile and lowers obesity risk.[38]

Pancreatic lipase: An enzyme for breaking down fats; take 30 minutes before a meal. When taken on an empty stomach, it helps fight cancer by stripping cancer cells of fibrin, an outer coating that shields them from your immune system.[39]

Ox bile: Essential bile salts for those with low bile production or without a gallbladder.

Collinsonia root (stone root): A herb used for centuries to remove gallstones and prevent constipation related to bile salt supplementation.

Chlorophyll: Humans and animals are photoheterotrophs, meaning we are able to use light for energy. Chlorophyll goes into the mitochondria as a metabolite and energizes them to produce more ATP (adenosine triphosphate), and hence more energy, without increasing oxidative stress.

Artichokes: Artichokes are a fabulous bile-producing food and liver protectant. Leaves from the artichoke plant contain caffeoylquinic acid, which promotes bile flow. Artichokes may boost glutathione levels as much as 50 percent.

Hydrochloric acid equivalents: Apple cider vinegar, lemon juice, or betaine HCl will boost stomach acid and stimulate bile and other digestive juices.

Dandelion root: Helps decrease liver congestion and increases bile flow due to a compound called taraxacin.

Vitamin C: A German study found that taking vitamin C daily can cut your risk of gallstones by nearly half.[40] Liposomal vitamin C is the most absorbable form; 1,000 to 5,000 milligrams per day is recommended.

THE BENEFITS OF INTERMITTENT FASTING

Overeating is the number one cause of gallbladder attacks, regardless of the type of food ingested. The stomach needs to be able to churn to mix your food with digestive juices—bile, stomach acid, and digestive enzymes. If your stomach is stuffed to the gills, it's like an overloaded washing machine—the clothes can't get clean. Food will be incompletely broken down, which means the nutrients will not be fully extracted and larger food particles pass into the bloodstream (leaky gut), setting you up for inflammation. Try this: for one week, reduce your portion sizes by half and see how you feel. If you're a habitual snacker, try eliminating snacks to allow your digestive system to rest and recover between workouts—you may be surprised at how much better you feel!

If you want to go a step further, intermittent fasting is another good strategy because it takes stress off your digestive system (including your liver and gallbladder), allowing it to rest and rejuvenate. When fasting, your body relearns how to burn fat as a primary fuel, as opposed to sugars. When fats are used for fuel, your liver manufactures water-soluble fats called ketones that burn more efficiently than carbohydrates. Burning ketones creates fewer free radicals that damage your cellular and mitochondrial cell membranes, proteins, and DNA. Training your body to efficiently burn fats improves glucose metabolism, reduces inflammation, and improves just about every aspect of your health. Intermittent fasting even protects the brain. This is the reason Ketogenic diets are often very successful—*as long as you can digest fats, that is.*

Science shows intermittent fasting lowers blood sugar and insulin levels and decreases insulin resistance, which facilitates loss of body fat—especially belly fat.[41] Intermittent fasting optimizes mitochondrial function and enhances important cellular repair processes, such as purging cellular waste,[42] which reduces oxidative stress and lowers inflammation.

One type of intermittent fasting is alternate day fasting, where you eat without restrictions one day, then consume about 500 calories the next. In one study, women practicing this style of fasting for eight weeks lost an average of 6kg. Science also indicates those who exercise in the morning on an empty stomach burn 20 percent more fat.[43] Kris Gunnars has a helpful beginner's guide to intermittent fasting.[44]

COFFEE ENEMAS AND THE TRADITIONAL GALLBLADDER FLUSH

Coffee enemas can be a powerful way to reduce your body's toxicity. Their benefits come from stimulation of the liver, more than the intestine—but they really have benefits for the entire body. Coffee enemas can help heal your digestive tract, relieve chronic pain, boost energy and mood, help eliminate parasites, and increase your liver's glutathione production. For further information, read *Achieve Maximum Health* by my friend and colleague David Webster, about the importance of colon hydrotherapy to overall health.

I would be remiss if I didn't mention the traditional gallbladder flush. The flush is a way to dissolve and flush out gallstones by using a combination of natural agents. Several liver/gallbladder flushes (sometimes called purges) are circulating on the Internet. I recommend avoiding these flushes because they can precipitate a life-threatening gallstone crisis. A stone that is blocked and unable to pass can create a medical emergency—which is exactly what you are trying to prevent!

IF YOU MUST PART WITH YOUR GALLBLADDER

I have seen many cases of serious gallbladder disease—including gallstones—being reversed using the strategies in this chapter. There is no downside to trying! Healing doesn't happen overnight, but many experience a relatively rapid abatement of symptoms. Everyone is different, but you can expect complete healing to take *at least* three to six months.

With proper support, many ailing gallbladders can heal, but sometimes the damage is too great and surgery is necessary—particularly in the case of a life-threatening infection. Whether you've had gallbladder surgery or not, the great news is that you don't have to shun fats for the rest of your life! A combination of bitters, bile salts, and the other ingredients and supplements listed in this chapter will accelerate your healing. If you do require surgery, you will probably need bile salts for a while (unless you have diarrhea or dumping syndrome). Even better is to supplement with both bile salts *and* bitters. Bile salts are more of a bile replacement, whereas bitters get your liver producing more bile so that in time you won't need to take bile salt replacements. Be mindful that, after you've healed, if you return to the same diet and lifestyle that produced the problem in the first place, then you'll be heading for trouble again, so in this respect it is a lifelong program. Bitter foods and bile-building foods should be permanent additions to your diet.

LET'S REVIEW

This chapter is really loaded with information, so let's connect a few dots. Your gall-bladder and bile are essential for fat digestion and absorption. And as you have learned, fats are vital to your health in every imaginable way. Bile is critical for preparing those life-sustaining omega-6 and omega-3 fats for incorporation into your cell membranes. If you give your gallbladder a little love by keeping your bile thin and free-flowing, your body will reward you by keeping your metabolism high and your toxin levels low, and by making sure your hormones play nicely together. On the other hand, if your bile becomes toxic, you increase your risk of a host of health problems from weight gain to low thyroid, estrogen dominance, body toxicity, and rampant inflammation.

Now that you're eating—and digesting—those healthy fats, in the next chapter, we'll shift our focus from fats to proteins.

4 RADICAL RULE # 3: REBUILD YOUR MUSCLES

Sometimes you don't realize your own strength until you come face to face with your greatest weaknesses.

—Susan Gale

IN THIS CHAPTER, YOU'LL LEARN . . .

- The skinny on why protein is critical
- How muscle is a metabolically active tissue that can rescue or ruin your weight-loss efforts
- Why muscle is the ultimate calorie burner
- The role of amino acids in providing energy, building muscle, and banishing cravings
- Which protein-rich foods will turn you into a lean, mean, fat-burning machine

It's time to power up your muscles! The best way to achieve this is to consume plenty of high-quality proteins every day. In Chapter 2, you learned how brown fat is the first of three key metabolically active tissues needed for a Radical Metabolism. Muscle is the second. Protein is to muscle tissue what dietary fat is to brown fat.

Muscle, like brown fat, is an innate ready-made energy burner. In fact, for every pound of muscle tissue, you will burn 50 calories per day, whereas each pound of body fat burns only a measly 2 calories! The greater your muscle mass, the more energy you will burn and the less fat you will store. It follows that the leaner you become, the easier it is to *stay* that way.

It's true: thinner people (those with a higher muscle-to-fat ratio) have a higher metabolic rate than do people with more body fat, so they burn more calories each day, even at rest. This can be you!

Just as brown fat is nourished and activated by the omega-6 fats in your diet, muscle is fueled by protein—amino acids, to be more precise. Like biological Lego, amino acids are building blocks that can be disassembled and reassembled into all the important proteins your body needs. When you "feed" your muscles, they return the favor by keeping you radically lean and healthy. Protein triggers fat burning and muscle building. It also helps stabilize your insulin and blood sugar levels, maintain energy, melt off body fat, and stave off the crave.

Protein's roles extend well beyond metabolism. The average body is about 20 percent protein by weight and contains an astounding 100,000 different proteins, all playing different roles. Proteins are used to make everything from muscles and vital organs to hormones and enzymes. Proteins also play an important role in detoxification—helping transport waste to your liver.

If your metabolism is on shaky ground, you might not be getting the right amount of protein in your meals each day, or not the right *combination* of proteins. Getting enough dietary protein spares lean body mass so that your body can burn fat for fuel. When you don't get adequate protein, your body begins breaking down its lean body mass for energy, as well as harvesting the amino acids it needs for routine tissue repairs. Not only does it obtain these proteins from your skeletal muscles but also from your organs—including your heart muscle. Unfortunately, when people diet they often wind up with *less muscle mass* than they started with—and of course this is the last thing you want. Your muscle cells shed proteins every day that your body must replace.

Low-calorie diets tend to alter the hormonal signals that stimulate muscle building. When dieting, your body is less likely to use the free amino acids in your bloodstream for muscle growth and repair, particularly if protein intake is too low.

Loss of lean body mass can be minimized by eating protein at every meal and making sure you're getting all the essential amino acids, which we'll talk about in this chapter. In addition to dietary protein, strength training and weight-bearing exercises, especially high-intensity, are very beneficial for building and maintaining lean body mass.

When you eat a quality protein-rich meal instead of a carb-heavy one, you're already ahead of the game in terms of energy expenditure. You actually burn more energy digesting protein than carbohydrates, even though they both contain the same calories (4 calories per gram). Twenty to thirty-five of every one hundred protein calories are burned up in the digestive process (this is known as the thermic effect).

Protein also benefits your blood sugar. Unlike when you eat carbohydrates, protein stimulates the release of glucagon, a hormone that helps you burn previously stored fat. Glucagon has the opposite effect of insulin and inhibits its release. It causes your body to *release* stored carbohydrates and fat, whereas insulin tells your body to *store* it. By eating protein throughout the day, you are keeping your body in glucagon-production mode.

All things considered, to optimize your metabolism you must consume enough high-quality protein. However, beware of overshooting the mark.

HOW MUCH PROTEIN SHOULD YOU BE EATING?

Protein is vital, but the truth is that problems can arise from consuming either *too much* or *too little*. Each of us has a sweet spot for protein intake.

Protein deficiency can manifest in a variety of conditions, such as sluggish metabolism, weight gain, loss of muscle mass, unstable blood sugars, insomnia and fatigue, mood swings, slow wound healing, and impaired immunity.

However, eating too much protein is hard on the kidneys. Protein is easy to overconsume on low-carb diets, such as Atkins and Ketogenic.

The body can only utilize 115–170g of protein at a time. Excess protein stresses the kidneys and liver, which must work hard to get rid of it.

Myth: You can't have too much protein in your diet.

The excess is metabolized into glucose and stored as body fat. If protein excess is extreme, your body can build up ammonia, a toxic waste product that can cause dangerous brain swelling, if levels become high enough. Excess protein also stimulates something called the mammalian target of rapamycin (mTOR) pathway, which accelerates aging and raises cancer risk. We'll be talking a bit more about mTOR later in this chapter.

Keep in mind, too, that even if you're overconsuming protein, it doesn't mean you're getting *optimal protein*. We get far too many low-quality proteins from processed foods and toxic factory-farmed animals. If your body can't use it, it doesn't count.

Given the risks associated with eating either too much or too little protein, what is the "Goldilocks zone"?

Each of us is unique in terms of our exact protein requirements due to such factors as age, gender, body weight, activity level, and overall health. The US government's recommended daily minimum protein intake for adults is 56 grams for men and 46 grams for women.[1] This translates to about 0.36 grams of protein per pound of body weight, which I and most contemporary experts believe is quite insufficient for optimal health. In the past, my gold standard has been 1.0 gram of protein per every 2.2 pounds of body weight, which equates to 0.45 grams of protein per pound.

I generally concur with the US's Food and Nutrition Board of the National Research Council, which has the following protein guidelines. Keep in mind that these numbers represent bare minimums, *not the amount for optimal health*. Your requirements will be higher, even double, if you are very active, pregnant, ill, or recovering from a serious injury, and lower if you have a sedentary lifestyle. The best way to determine your ideal amount is by trial and error, with 1.5 grams per pound of body weight being the upper limit.

Adult men	70 grams
Adult women	58 grams
Pregnant women	65 grams
Lactating women	75 grams
Girls, aged 13–15	62 grams
Girls, aged 16–20	58 grams
Boys, aged 13–15	75 grams
Boys, aged 16–20	85 grams

We tend to lose more muscle mass with age (sarcopenia), so as we get older, our protein requirements may change. Declining muscle mass often begins earlier than you might think, typically in your thirties. With sarcopenia comes weight gain, insulin resistance, and metabolic syndrome that may progress to full-blown type 2 diabetes. There is also a strong relationship between muscle mass, strength, and overall function as we age—including falls. Brain injuries among adults age seventy-five and older have increased by 76 percent since 2007, and the primary cause is falling.[2] Sarcopenia correlates strongly with disability, poor quality of life, and earlier death—in other words, *lean body mass is crucial to your health and longevity*.

As we move into our elder years, our appetite may dwindle due to diminished taste and smell. Many seniors also become less active, accelerating their rate of muscle loss. Many will benefit from a high-quality protein drink, such as whey. Amino acid supplementation has been shown to improve body composition in people with muscle wasting illnesses, especially liver disease.[3]

PROTEINS FOR SKINNY JEANS

If you dream of getting back into those skinny jeans, then you must focus on consuming the right building blocks for muscle tissue. The best approach is to consume a clean, whole-food–based diet with a wide variety of foods. In terms of getting the highest-quality proteins, you'll want to avoid animal products from confined animal feeding operations, where livestock are fed an unnatural diet of GMO grains instead of fresh grass from pasture. Source your meats from organic, local farms that raise their animals on pasture with minimal grain-based feed, hormones, and agricultural chemicals.

Other good protein sources include wild fish, such as Pacific salmon, sardines, and anchovies; pasture-raised poultry and raw dairy; and nuts and seeds. Legumes can provide you with good (but not complete) proteins, but their complex carbohydrates can spike your insulin, so they're problematic for some. Hemp seeds boast more than 4 grams of protein per tablespoon, and pumpkin seeds have 2 grams per tablespoon. Spirulina also provides 4 grams of protein per tablespoon, and don't forget that wonderful tahini sporting 4 grams of protein in every tablespoon.

PROTEIN CONTENT OF FOODS

FOOD	PROTEIN CONTENT
Red meat, poultry, fish, seafood	6–9 grams per 30g
Hard cheeses	7–8 grams per 30g
Yogurt	17 grams per 170g
Seeds and nuts	1–2 grams per tablespoon
Hemp seeds	4.4 grams per tablespoon
Chia seeds	2.4 grams per tablespoon
Tahini	4 grams per tablespoon
Most cooked legumes	7–8 grams per 90g
Cooked lentils	18 grams per 200g
Cooked soybeans	28 grams per 170g
Most vegetables	1–2 grams per 30g
Cooked amaranth	7 grams per 250g
Cooked buckwheat	6 grams per 170g
Spirulina	4 grams per tablespoon

IS LOW STOMACH ACID ROBBING YOU OF PROTEIN?

Trouble digesting protein can make you protein deficient—and the main culprit is low stomach acid. Not only is adequate hydrochloric acid (HCl) necessary for fat digestion, but it's an absolute requirement for protein digestion. HCl is first on the scene to break down the larger protein pieces from your meal into long amino chains. Then, enzymes, such as protease and peptidase, finish the processing, with the end result being small peptides and free amino acids that are easily absorbed and usable by the body.

No matter how many high-quality proteins you eat, if your stomach acid is low (see page 14), you won't be able to break down those fabulous protein-rich foods into their essential amino acids. A diet too high in protein can also overwhelm HCl production.

The result? Body composition starts to tank. Your muscles shrink and you start stockpiling fat. The fact that we lose HCl production as we age is another reason we tend to lose muscle mass as we get older. Pancreatic proteolytic enzymes can be taken as a supplement, but better yet, they are found naturally in certain foods—for example, papaya, which contains the proteolytic enzyme papain.

AMINO ACIDS: THE MISSING LINK FOR WEIGHT LOSS

Proteins are key to a radical metabolism due to the amino acids they provide. Just as with *essential fatty acids*, your body must have the correct balance of *essential amino acids* to keep your metabolism abuzz.

You've already seen how eating protein accelerates your metabolism and encourages fat burning. If we don't consume enough protein, our bodies have no choice but to break down our muscles and organs to get the amino acids (and energy) they need.

Roughly three hundred types of amino acids occur in nature, but only twenty-two are used by the body—which is amazing when you consider it manages to make 100,000 different proteins out of these mere twenty-two!

Because proteins have so many functions, they are constantly being "repurposed" by your body, broken down, and replaced. They are disassembled into their component parts—the amino acid building blocks—and then reassembled into new forms in a complex process called protein biosynthesis. Your amino acids are recycled three to four times a day—so that chicken breast you ate for lunch may do a little time on your biceps, then get morphed into dopamine and serotonin, before being transformed into fuel by your liver!

Unlike fat and starch, the body does not store excess amino acids for later use (at least, not long term), so you must get them from your foods every day. Symptoms of amino acid deficiency depend on which aminos are missing, so vary widely.

Not only do the aminos serve as building blocks for your muscles and vital organs, but they also compose an assortment of other molecules, such as neurotransmitters and compounds that regulate your immune system. Amino acids enable vitamins and minerals to perform their functions, and form the base structures of DNA—the "backbone" of your chromosomes. As a component of enzymes, aminos play important roles in nearly all life-sustaining biological processes. Because amino acids are sensitive to pH, enzymes don't work properly unless your pH is correct.

Perhaps the most elemental function of amino acids is their use in cell membranes. Yes, my friends, we are back to those! Whereas phospholipids, those key fats we talked about in Chapter 2, provide the basic cell membrane structure, amino acids are used to build cellular substructures, such as transport channels and hormone receptors, as well as proteins that carry out biological tasks. Think of some as "runners" and "communicators."[4] For example, transporter proteins help usher other molecules, like glucose, in and out of the cell. Your body's mitochondrial membranes are 75 percent amino acids. It's estimated that a whopping 30 percent of our genes are devoted to encoding membrane proteins—which tells us just how important they are!

Most diseases, if not all, involve a breakdown in cellular communication. Cell-to-cell communication relies upon these protein elements, and if the right amino acids are not available to make them, then signals get scrambled.[5] This is what happens with metabolic malfunction, weight-loss resistance, hormone imbalance, diabetes . . . and the list goes on. (Toxicity also plays a major role in corrupting cell-to-cell dialogue, which we'll be covering in Chapter 6.) That's why getting the right complement of amino acids in your diet is so important.

WHAT CAN AMINOS DO FOR YOU?

Now let's look at a few specific amino acids and the highlights of what they can do for you, especially when it comes to reinvigorating a sluggish metabolism. (For information about the functions of all twenty-two and their food sources, please refer to the extensive table at the end of this chapter.)

Your body's twenty-two amino acids can be divided into three types: essential amino acids (EAAs), non-essential amino acids, and conditionally essential (sometimes called semi-essential) amino acids. *Essential* means your body does not make them, so it must get them from your diet. The non-essential aminos can be manufactured by your body, and the conditionally essential can be manufactured unless you are ill or stressed.

Foods that are "complete proteins" contain all ten essential amino acids. If you fail to get *even one* of the EAAs in your diet, then your body will need to break down muscle tissue to liberate it—which makes complete proteins a highly valuable part of your diet. Most complete proteins come from animal products. Although many plant foods are rich in multiple amino acids, the only complete proteins from the plant kingdom are soybeans, quinoa, buckwheat, chia seeds, hemp seeds, and spirulina.

AMINO ACIDS

ESSENTIAL AMINO ACIDS

Arginine	Histadine	Isoleucine
Leucine	Lysine	Methionine
Phenylalanine	Threonine	Tryptophan
Valine		

CONDITIONALLY ESSENTIAL AMINO ACIDS

Cysteine	Glutamine	Glycine
Ornithine	Proline	Serine
Taurine	Tyrosine	

NON-ESSENTIAL AMINO ACIDS

Alanine	Asparagine	Aspartate
Glutamate		

Each amino acid has its own special functions in the body. For example, *histidine* is used in the making of histamines, a key part of your immune response. *Threonine* is necessary for making the pigment in red blood cells that binds iron. *Valine* helps bind proteins together. *Lysine* boosts collagen production and kills viruses, and *tryptophan* helps us sleep.

In terms of weight loss—specifically, fat loss and muscle building—a few aminos may be of particular value: glutamine, lysine, methionine, phenylalanine, ornithine, leucine, isoleucine, and valine.

Glutamine helps reduce fat deposition, improves insulin signaling, and helps reduce sugar and alcohol cravings.

The liver combines the two EAAs *lysine* and *methionine* into *carnitine*, a prime fat burner. Carnitine is stored in muscle tissue, where it helps shuttle fatty acids into the cells' mitochondria for use in making adenosine triphosphate (ATP), which is fuel. This process is especially active during exercise.

Phenylalanine is a natural appetite suppressant.

Ornithine can make you leaner because it stimulates human growth hormone (HGH), when taken before bed (2,500 milligrams).

Leucine, isoleucine, and *valine*, which are branched-chain amino acids (BCAAs), work together in the muscle tissue assembly line. Let's talk a little more about these BCAAs.

BRANCHED-CHAIN AMINO ACIDS: THE AMINOS FOR YOUR MUSCLES

Some call branched-chain amino acids (BCAAs) the "missing link to weight loss." Leucine, isoleucine, and valine were given this name for their branched molecular structure. Whereas most amino acids are broken down in your liver, BCAAs are broken down mostly in your muscles, where they play important roles in energy, endurance, and maintenance of lean body mass.

BCAAs perform the following biological functions:

- They improve your endurance and reduce fatigue due to improving energy production (particularly isoleucine and valine).[6]
- They reduce muscle loss and increase muscle building (particularly leucine).[7]
- They increase fat metabolism, and decrease fat deposition.[8]
- They speed exercise recovery, reducing muscle soreness and spasms.[9]
- They have positive effects on blood glucose, insulin, and triglyceride levels (particularly isoleucine and valine).[10]

BCAAs comprise about 35 percent of all muscle tissue. If you don't have adequate BCAAs, your body will break down muscle tissue to obtain them, resulting in greater muscle loss. In other words, BCAAs help you preserve and build your lean body mass so that your body fuels itself with stored body fat instead of muscle. Although your liver can convert BCAAs into energy, the process is a little clunky, whereas your muscles are ready-made for the task! Estimates are that BCAAs provide 18 percent or more of your body's "workout fuel." Leucine is a particularly important BCAA for creating a lean body, due to its ability to stimulate muscle-building.

BCAAS ARE BEST OBTAINED FROM FOODS

The latest science suggests the minimum daily requirements for BCAAs are 9 grams per day for women and 12 grams per day for men, ideally from food, not supplements. People who get plenty of high-quality protein in their diets are unlikely to need supplements. You can obtain BCAAs from protein-rich foods, such as organic grass-pastured beef and dairy, wild Alaskan salmon, nuts, and seeds. (For sources unique to each amino, see the table at the end of this chapter.)

If you happen to be an athlete or engaged in heavy resistance training, or if you are vegan or vegetarian, a daily supplement might be beneficial, in the dose of 10 to 20 grams of BCAAs. The best time to take these is before and/or after a workout. We need 8 to 16 grams of leucine daily for optimal muscle growth and repair.

Whey protein is an excellent source of all the EAAs, especially leucine—85g of whey protein provide 8 grams of leucine compared to 1.6 grams in 85g of salmon, for example. When it comes to muscle building, whey protein may out-perform BCAA supplements.[11] Besides being rich in leucine, whey protein has sixty-four different amino acids that perform a symphony of functions, including appetite suppression. Whey is a potent stimulator of cholecystokinin (CCK), *the hormone that stimulates bile release*. In one study, whey increased CCK more than 400 percent.[12]

As long as you are consuming the right kind, whey protein has a mountain of benefits, especially for your immune system, including fighting cancer. Whey also has anti-inflammatory, antioxidant, blood pressure-lowering and stress-reducing proper-ties. However, many people are consuming whey products containing inferior quality whey that not only lacks immune benefits but can actually trigger allergies and other problems.

There are two kinds of milk from which whey products are made: A1 and A2 beta-casein. The majority are made from A1 milk, which is mutated and associated with allergies, digestive problems, cardiovascular issues, and diabetes. You want your whey derived from A2 milk because it's non-mutated and cold processed to preserve the delicate protein and amino acid structures. Unfortunately, most cow's milk in North America is A1. Make sure your whey products are free of GMOs, hormones, gluten, excess sugar, chemical additives, and, of course, heavy metal contamination.

It's been said that the initial 40 grams of protein you consume each day specifi-cally target your immune system—so make them count!

MAPS: PROTEIN IN A PILL

If you choose to supplement with amino acids, a cutting edge new product enjoys many advantages over the other amino acid supplements. MAP, short for "master amino pattern," provides eight essential amino acids in a highly purified, free, crystal-line form. This is just about as close to "Star Trek nutrition" as you can get! MAP is digested very rapidly—within 23 minutes—because it doesn't require the aid of stom-ach acid or pancreatic enzymes. MAP is also virtually acaloric. Studies show 99 percent of MAP is utilized immediately by the body to make proteins, which beats dietary proteins that have only 16 to 48 percent utilization. MAPS are typically taken like BCAAs, shortly before or after a workout. They can also be used by vegans to increase daily protein, in three-times-a-day dosing.

CAUTIONS ABOUT SUPPLEMENTATION

BCAA supplements are not without some potential side effects, which is why I sug-gest getting your amino acids from your foods. Our bodies are the masters when it comes to balancing the amino acids properly and in the right ratios. As you'll recall, amino acids are used to make chemical messengers, and mucking around with neurotransmitters and hormones and such may have unintended consequences under certain conditions. The effects can vary, depending on your diet and other lifestyle factors.

For example, BCAAs may either decrease blood sugar levels or raise them, depending on the circumstances. Some studies have found using BCAA supplements while on a high-fat diet can lead to insulin resistance and type 2 diabetes.[13] Both diabetes and cancer are characterized by dysfunctional cell signaling, so caution must be exercised with anything that alters how cells communicate.[14]

Another concern about amino acid supplementation is stimulation of the mTOR pathway. MTOR decides whether cells should replicate now or wait for a more opportune time. Amino acids are the *most potent stimulators* of mTOR. If you have excess aminos, then mTOR becomes upregulated (stimulated), which can accelerate aging. Virtually all cancers are associated with mTOR stimulation.[15] What you want is for mTOR to be downregulated (suppressed) because this promotes maintenance and repair and increases longevity. *The bottom line is, don't overdo or underdo your protein!*

AMINO ACID FUNCTIONS AND FOOD SOURCES

AMINO ACID	FUNCTIONS	FOOD SOURCES
Arginine	Nitrogen retention and nitric acid production for healthy blood flow, oxygenation, and blood pressure; stimulates HGH (human growth hormone); muscle synthesis; necessary for creatine (energy source for muscles); collagen; essential for children up to age 5 and adults above age 60	Alfalfa sprouts, beetroots, carrots, celery, chicken breast, chickpeas, cucumbers, dairy, green vegetables, leeks, lentils, lettuce, nutritional yeast, parsnips, potatoes, pumpkin seeds, radishes, soybeans, turkey
Histidine	Nerve transmission and myelin sheaths; synthesis of histamine; blood pressure support; essential for children up to age 5	Alfalfa sprouts, apples, beef, beetroots, bison, carrots, celery, chicken, cucumbers, dandelion greens, endive, fish, garlic, pomegranates, radish, spinach, turkey, turnip greens
Leucine	(BCAA) Muscle energy; protein synthesis; strong potentiator of HGH; exercise recovery; tissue healing; insulin and glucose utilization; decreases visceral fat; healing after injury; muscle sparing	Avocado, beans, beef, cheese, chicken, coconut, fish, nuts, olives, papaya, seafood, seeds, soybeans, whey

AMINO ACID FUNCTIONS AND FOOD SOURCES

AMINO ACID	FUNCTIONS	FOOD SOURCES
Isoleucine	(BCAA) Blood sugar regulation and energy stabilization; stimulates HCG release; muscle healing and repair; hemoglobin; clotting; primary defense against infection through open wounds	Alfalfa sprouts, avocado, cheese, chicken, coconut, crustaceans, fish, game meats, olives, bok choy, papaya, pheasant, seaweed, spinach, sunflower seeds, Swiss chard, turkey, watercress
Lysine	Collagen and elastin; component of fat-burner, mitochondrial-booster carnitine; boosts calcium uptake for bone building	Alfalfa sprouts, apples, apricots, beans, beetroots, carrots, celery, cheese, chicken, cucumber, dandelion greens, fish, grapes, beef, lentils, nuts, papaya, parsley, pears, seeds, shellfish, soybeans, spinach, turkey, turnip greens
Methionine	Sulfur for synthesis of hemoglobin and glutathione; component of fat-burner, mitochondrial-booster carnitine; cartilage, hair and nails	Apples, beans, beef, Brazil nuts, cabbage, cauliflower, cheese, chives, dairy, filberts (hazelnuts), fish, garlic, horseradish, kale, pineapple, shellfish, sorrel, soybeans, turkey, watercress
Phenylalanine	Precursor to catecholamines (regulation of nervous system); stimulates cholecystokinin (CCK) for bile release and satiation; best avoided if you are pregnant or have hypertension, phenylketonuria, melanoma, anxiety attacks, or take MAO inhibitors	Almonds, apples, avocados, bananas, beetroots, carrots, cheese, fish, butter beans, nutritional yeast, parsley, pineapple, pumpkin seeds, sesame seeds, soybeans, spinach, tomatoes
Threonine	Synthesis of porphyrin for binding iron; collagen and elastin; digestive enzymes; antibody production and thymus gland; liver function; increases bioavailability of other nutrients	Alfalfa sprouts, beans, carrots, celery, cheese, chicken, green leafy vegetables, beef, lentils, lettuce, liver, nori, nuts, papaya, seeds, shellfish, soy
Tryptophan	Reduces stress, promotes sleep; growth and development; precursor to serotonin and melatonin; niacin	Alfalfa sprouts, beans, Brussels sprouts, carrots, celery, cheese, chicken, chives, dandelion greens, endive (chicory), fennel, fish, lentils, nutritional yeast, nuts, oats, red meat, seeds, green beans, spinach, tofu, turkey, turnips
Valine	(BCAA) Treatment of liver and gallbladder disorders; glycogen synthesis; insulin secretion; binds proteins together; regulates absorption of other amino acids; mental acuity	Almonds, apples, beans, beef, beetroots, celery, cheese, chicken, dandelion greens, fish, lettuce, mushrooms, nutritional yeast, nuts, okra, parsley, parsnips, pomegranates, seeds, soybeans, squash, tomatoes, turnips
Cysteine	An unstable sulfur molecule (quickly converts to cystine); required for glutathione synthesis so critical for detox; blood pressure and blood sugar stabilization	Beef, cheese, chicken, fish, legumes, oats, soybeans, sunflower seeds
Glycine	Provides glucose for muscle; regulates blood sugar; bile production; energy production; collagen; hemoglobin; blood pressure; DNA building block; required for creatine synthesis; wound healing; calms central nervous system so may help panic attacks; hormone balance; epilepsy	Beef, chicken, mollusks, ostrich, sesame seeds, spinach, watercress

AMINO ACID	FUNCTIONS	FOOD SOURCES
Glutamine	Counters fat deposition; improves insulin signaling and glucose; reduces blood glucose and cravings (easily converts to glucose); reduces lactic acid; facilitates healing by building fibroblasts and epithelial cells; gut maintenance and repair; passes through blood–brain barrier; neurotransmitter for memory and focus; blood pressure; increases HGH; nitrogen detox and ammonia reduction; DNA building block; most abundant amino acid in the body (60 percent of pool)	Asparagus, bone broth, broccoli rabe (rapini), Chinese cabbage, cottage cheese, beef, spirulina, turkey, venison, fish
Proline	Collagen; builds strong blood vessels to combat arteriosclerosis and stabilize blood pressure	Asparagus, beef, broccoli rabe (rapini), cabbage, cheese, chicken, chives, gelatin, watercress
Serine	Brain and central nervous system; myelin sheaths; phospholipids; fatty acid metabolism; DNA and RNA function; helps produce immunoglobulins and antibodies; creatine absorption	Baby squash, bamboo shoots, bison, cottage cheese, cream cheese, cuttlefish, elk, kidney beans, pike, quail, seaweed, turkey breast, watercress
Tyrosine	Synthesis of noradrenaline, dopamine, and thyroid hormones; improves memory under stress	Beans, beef, cheese, chicken, dairy, fish, kidney beans, mustard greens, nuts, seeds, soybeans, spinach, turnip greens, watercress
Taurine	Promotes bile acids and thins the bile; detoxes heavy metals; boosts metabolism; decreases liver fat; heart and brain health; activates GABA	Chicken (dark meat), dairy, fish, meat, nutritional yeast, organ meats (offal), seaweed, shellfish
Ornithine	Converts to arginine; helps ammonia convert to urea and clear from the bloodstream; stimulates HGH (human growth hormone); also see arginine	See arginine
Alanine	Synthesized from lactic acid by muscle cells; very important for blood glucose regulation; reduces fatigue by boosting carnosine	Beef, fish, parsley, poultry, soybeans, sunflower seeds, white mushrooms
Asparagine	Balance and equilibrium; nerve function; used in large number of proteins	Asparagus, dairy, fish, legumes, nuts, potatoes, poultry, red meat, soybeans
Aspartate	(Aspartic acid) Metabolism; ATP; synthesis of other amino acids; mental sharpness; ammonia detox	Asparagus, bamboo shoots, cod, crab, lentils, mung beans, peppers, spinach, tuna, white fish
Glutamate	Most common neurotransmitter in brain and spinal cord; synthesis of GABA (natural calming agent); energy; blood pressure; immune and digestive support	Avocados, beans, chicken breast, dairy, fish, kelp, lentils, lobster, red meat, poultry, salmon, sunflower seeds, turkey breast, wakame, walnuts

1.   Fred Pescatore, *The A-List Diet: Lose up to 15 Pounds and Look And Feel Younger in Just 2 Weeks* (Dallas, TX: BenBella Books, Inc., 2017).

CARNITINE FOR A METABOLIC BOOST

Carnitine is an amino acid "cousin" found in nearly every cell in your body; it helps your mitochondria metabolize and eliminate fat. Studies also suggest that carnitine may improve thyroid function. Carnitine is the generic name for a number of compounds, including L-carnitine and acetyl-L-carnitine.

Carnitine plays a critical role in energy production by transporting long-chain fatty acids into the mitochondria so they can be oxidized ("burned") for energy, then escorts toxic compounds out of the cell. Carnitine also protects your liver from noxious agents. As we age, carnitine stores often become depleted. Swiss scientists have shown that early carnitine deficiencies may result in liver problems and loss of glycogen stores in muscle tissue.[16]

Given the fact that it is used by tissues that utilize fatty acids for fuel, carnitine is most concentrated in your skeletal and cardiac muscle, where it can facilitate energy metabolism and exercise endurance. That said, acetyl-L-carnitine is also beneficial for memory by revving up energy-depleted brain cells.

TAKING THE WORK OUT OF YOUR WORKOUTS

We all know the importance of regular exercise, but the latest research has become laser focused on the dangers of prolonged sitting. *Sitting is the new smoking.* It used to be believed that going to the gym was enough to counter the effects of a sedentary job, but this has not proved true. Prolonged sitting is linked to heart disease, diabetes, and premature death—even among those who exercise up to an hour per day.[17] Scientists aren't sure exactly how sitting causes so many problems for your body, but some studies indicate it's related to altered sugar and fat metabolism. This says to me that excessive sitting is a great way to snuff out a radical metabolism!

The key to minimizing the damage from sitting is to move intermittently throughout your day. Avoid sitting for more than thirty minutes at a time, even if you get up only briefly—one to three minutes at a time is all you need. We burn 30 percent more calories when standing than when sitting. This is why standing desks have become so popular. Make standing your first new habit!

In addition to getting up from your chair more often, there are many ways to increase your daily activity level. One of my favorites is simply taking a walk, especially in nature. It's easy, you can do it pretty much anywhere, and the price is right. Rebounding is another fabulous exercise that also improves lymphatic flow, which helps detoxification.

Whether you're going for forest walks or doing yoga, Tai Chi, aerobics classes, or whatever, the best approach is to vary your activity as much as possible and select activities you actually enjoy. If you're not having fun, the odds of your sticking to it are pretty bleak. Ideally, your activities should include short bursts of high-intensity work, weight-bearing and resistance exercise, stretching, balance, and flexibility—and a little *rest* so that you don't overdo it.

To recap, in this chapter you've learned how to harness the power of protein to flip on your fat-burning/muscle-building switches. Consuming a full range of amino acids, including those muscle-friendly BCAAs, along with increasing your daily activity, will go a long way toward returning you to the lean and lively person you remember! The next step is to radically improve your digestive tract.

5 RADICAL RULE #4: REPAIR YOUR GUT

Natural forces within us are the true healers of disease.

—Hippocrates

IN THIS CHAPTER, YOU'LL LEARN . . .

- How your gut flora, or microbiome, can keep you lean and healthy
- Do you have skinny bugs or fat bugs?
- How metabolic mayhem can be triggered by gluten, lectins, and other foods
- Why a leaky gut can inhibit weight loss and fat burning, increase "false fat," and more
- 7 simple strategies to keep you slim with a happy, healthy gut

If you've been reading anything lately about diet and nutrition, I'm sure this chapter will not come as a surprise. The truth is, if you are constantly fighting your weight, feeling stressed, or your bowels are always backed up, then you probably have a messy microbiome.

Think of your microbiome as another organ, one that plays a role in nearly every process in your body—including your metabolism. You have already learned how brown fat and muscle tissue are two metabolically active tissues. *And now you have the third: the microbiome!*

Each of us carries around a diverse community of microscopic life on and within our bodies—trillions of microorganisms playing together in one giant symphony. A large segment of your microbiome resides in your digestive tract, and this microbial community is involved in everything from your digestion to your immune function, emotions, and behavior. They might even be controlling those carbohydrate cravings . . . you could be eating to satisfy a hungry horde! Science has shown that our food preferences, energy use, fat storage, and body composition are heavily influenced by the types of bacteria that live in our guts.

But here is where it gets messy.

The foods you eat, your daily stresses, sleep, toxic exposures, medications, and other factors all work together to alter your microbiome, *for better or for worse*. Your digestive tract may be harboring mostly "skinny bugs" . . . or mostly "fat bugs"!

More than two thousand years ago, Hippocrates, long regarded as the "father of medicine," stated that "all disease begins in the gut"—and now an explosion of science proves he was right. Our bodies have evolved a symbiotic relationship with the microbial world. Your gut flora occupies every square centimeter of your digestive tract from your mouth to your anus, each region housing a unique community of microorganisms (mainly bacteria, but also viruses, fungi, and protozoa[1]) that have adapted to those specific conditions and perform functions for your benefit. For example, more than six hundred species of bacteria have been identified in the mouth alone, with healthy population counts required for prevention of cavities, throat and ear infections, and even halitosis. Friendly gut bacteria (especially certain strains of *Bifidobacteria*) synthesize B vitamins for us, including B_{12}, folate, biotin, thiamine, and niacin. Behind the scenes, these tiny organisms are also epigenetic superheroes, influencing our cells' genetic expression—whether certain genes are activated—including genes affecting your body weight.

If you have a healthy, balanced microbiome, around 85 percent of your bacteria will be the beneficial variety and only 15 percent pathogenic. However, if too many of the wrong microbes take over and this ratio goes upside down (dysbiosis), your immunity, cellular communication, and metabolism can tumble like dominos.

Although every individual's microbiome is unique, like fingerprints, science is discovering that certain diseases have unique microbial signatures. The makeup of your microbiome is continuously changing in response to shifts in diet, lifestyle, stress, and exposure to toxic agents. Several factors are known to shape your microbiome throughout your life, from the type of birth you had (vaginal or Caesarean) to your diet as a baby (breast milk or formula), your diet as an adult, frequency of antibiotic use, and chemical exposures.

The typical modern-day diet and lifestyle inflict a lot of damage on our native flora. Refined sugar, artificial sweeteners, certain sugar alcohols, chemicals, and processed foods deal serious blows to your friendly flora. Gluten, the protein found in wheat, rye, and barley, is particularly problematic as well, even for those who do not consider themselves to be gluten sensitive. Poor sleep habits, inactivity, and chronic stress further contribute to a messy microbiome.

The good news? The microbiome's plasticity means you can restore it with a few basic strategies, and the resultant health benefits will quickly trickle upstream. If a radically improved metabolism is what you're going for, then keeping your microbiome happy and healthy is a top priority.

Myth: Bacteria outnumber human cells 10:1 in the human body.

HOW MANY BACTERIA DO WE HAVE, ANYWAY?

This oft-cited but exaggerated statistic has been in circulation for many years, originating in 1972 with microbiologist Thomas Lucky who reportedly never intended that his estimate be widely quoted decades later. Current calculations using a more sophisticated sampling methodology place the real number closer to 1.3:1 bacterial cells to human cells.[2] The latest estimate for the total number of human cells in our bodies is 37.2 trillion,[3] for a ballpark figure of 48 trillion bacteria per person. *That's still a lot of bacteria!*

In a healthy gut, friendly bacteria number around 100 billion to 1,000 billion per millimeter of digestive tract. Americans have been found to house as few as *five organisms per millimeter*—with the remainder all being unfriendly bugs. No wonder so many people are struggling with their weight, digestion, and hormones!

YOUR MICROBIOME MATTERS FOR WEIGHT, HORMONES, AND HEALTH

We carry an impressive bacterial load, but what our single-celled companions *do* for us is even more impressive! Your gut flora informs everything from your bowel habits to cancer risk. When it comes to appetite, blood sugar stability, synthesis of nutrients, and even detox, your microbiome is calling the shots.

If you become a host to large colonies of the wrong bacteria, the health effects can be profound. They can trigger disease by flipping undesirable genes into the ON position. Altered microbiomes are associated with a mind-numbing array of conditions, such as Parkinson's disease, chronic fatigue, bowel disorders (Crohn's disease, IBD, and IBS), skin ailments, and many more.[4] Sometimes the role these organisms play is very basic. For example, your microbiome can protect you from heart attack and stroke because these friendly flora are one of your best sources of carotenoids.[5]

HOW YOUR GUT FLORA KEEPS YOU HEALTHY

DIGESTION, METABOLISM, BODY WEIGHT & COMPOSITION	IMMUNITY, HORMONES, DETOX & OTHER
Digestion and absorption	Immune health and control of pathogens through "competitive exclusion"
Synthesis of nutrients (B vitamins, carotenoids, vitamin K, enzymes, CLA, folic acid, vitamin D)	Modulation of inflammation (limitation of cytokine production)
Optimal use of antioxidants, including polyphenols	Detoxification
Mineral bioavailability	Deactivation of cancer-causing compounds
Amino acid metabolism	Optimal liver function
Appetite control	Hormone regulation
Blood sugar stability	Stress reduction (by regulating stress hormones, cortisol and adrenalin)
Healthy body weight and prevention of obesity	Mental health and positive moods (synthesis of serotonin and other neurotransmitters, gut–brain connection)
Carbohydrate absorption	Lipid metabolism and cholesterol regulation
Bile acid recycling	Pain control
Lactase production (an enzyme required for digestion of dairy)	Sleep quality
Healthy gut barrier	Longevity
Normalization of bowel movements	

FAT BACTERIA, SKINNY BACTERIA

Is an unbalanced microbiome increasing your waistline?

Two factors have a profound impact on metabolism: microbial diversity, and the ratio of *Firmicutes* to *Bacteroidetes* bacteria in your gut. Belgian professor Patrice D. Cani discovered that obesity is associated with reduced numbers of certain species of gut bacteria from the phylum *Bacteroidetes* and increased numbers from certain species in the phylum *Firmicutes*. He is also investigating the use of the bacterial species *Akkermansia muciniphila* as a treatment for obesity because people with greater numbers of those organisms appear to have a stronger metabolism, lower inflammation, and better intestinal function.[6]

Studies show that lean individuals have more diverse microbiomes than overweight individuals, and people with more diverse microbiomes live longer.[7] As diversity declines, opportunistic pathogens take over, which stresses the body and drives up inflammation, food cravings, weight gain, diabetes risk, mood instability, hormone dysfunction, and a host of other problems that add misery to your life while carving years off your life span.

Firmicutes and *Bacteroidetes* make up 90 percent of the bacteria in your colon. *Firmicutes* are "fat-loving" bacteria that are extremely proficient at extracting calories from food, which increases fat absorption. These guys lead you down the road toward obesity, diabetes, and heart disease. On the other side of the ring are *Bacteroidetes*, which specialize in breaking down plant starches and fibers into energy your body can use, in the form of shorter-chain fatty acids. A study from Washington University showed that obese individuals have 20 percent more *Firmicutes* and 90 percent fewer *Bacteroidetes*, on average. A simple way to improve your ratio is by consuming more fiber.

On the other hand, two bacterial strains, *Lactobacillus rhamnosus* and *Lactobacillus gasseri*, are on the radar for offering special benefits to those needing to lose weight. In a 2014 study, women taking the *rhamnosus* strain experienced significant reductions in fat mass as well as drops in circulating leptin levels (effectively decreasing appetite), with benefits continuing even after supplementation was discontinued.[8] *Lactobacillus gasseri* was shown to reduce weight and waist and hip circumference for obese and overweight adults.[9] Yet another species, *Bacillus coagulans*, appears to be very proficient at inactivating lectins. (You will be learning about the adverse effects of lectins later in this chapter.)

Healthy gut bacteria also increase bile production and help regulate your cholesterol levels. Yes, we're back to that all-important bile! In your colon, they convert primary bile acids into secondary bile acids, which improves reabsorption rates. About 95 percent of bile should be recycled, meaning it should be reabsorbed through intestinal walls and returned to the liver. On the other hand, pathogenic bacteria convert bile acids into the toxic compound lithocholate, which interferes with your liver's ability to convert cholesterol into bile acids, driving cholesterol levels up. Bile also increases the survival rate of the good bacteria in your colon while suppressing the bad.

Your microbiome is not limited to bacteria—fungi play a role as well, which is referred to as your mycobiome. Scientists have discovered that fungal populations are also distinctly different between lean and overweight individuals, although the details are still being investigated.[10] Certain parasitic infections can affect metabolism as well, which I cover in my book *Guess What Came to Dinner?*

THE HORMONE CONNECTION

Your microbiome profoundly influences your hormone status. When you have dysbiosis (too many pathogenic organisms), you will experience appetite changes because those pathogens dramatically influence your hunger hormones.

There really is no separation between you and your microbiome. You can almost consider them as another body organ—they have that much control over your physiology. Their survival is completely dependent on your diet, so they have devised mechanisms to control you (their "host") through something called gut-brain signaling. To get their needs met and ensure their survival, they produce molecules (neuropeptides) that directly affect your brain, particularly the hypothalamus, as that's your hunger and satiety center.[11] In other words, they hijack your hormone system and try to make you their food slave.

Estrogen is another example of how your microbiome affects your hormone status. Up to 60 percent of circulating estrogen is normally picked up by your liver and "deactivated" before being dumped into your gallbladder, where it's trapped in the bile and excreted through the bowel. Beneficial bacteria produce an enzyme that reactivates estrogen so it can be reabsorbed by the body. When your microbiome is off-kilter, this recycling doesn't occur so you lose more estrogen in your stool. Low estrogen levels are associated with osteoporosis, PMS, migraines, water retention, and other problems. A similar mechanism has been suggested with several other hormones, as well as folic acid, vitamin B_{12}, cholesterol, and vitamin D.

Digestive disorders and hormone problems go hand in hand. Estrogen and progesterone influence digestion, which may be why digestive disorders are more common among women. Problems tend to be worse during the latter half of the menstrual cycle (luteal phase) when transit time slows, with a sharp rise in digestive complaints just before the onset of menses. Women also report a digestive slowdown during menopause and premenopause.

THE GUT–BRAIN CONNECTION

Have you ever had "butterflies" in your stomach or experienced an episode of diarrhea from extreme performance anxiety? This is your "second brain" talking to you. There is a major connection between your gut and your brain. In your gut resides the enteric nervous system (ENS), which senses and reacts to any perceived threat. Like a red phone to the Oval Office, signals travel from your gut to your brain along the vagus nerve. This is referred to as the gut-brain axis. Just like the brain, the enteric nervous system utilizes more than thirty neurotransmitters. At last, those gut feelings are being explained by science!

Studies suggest that alteration of the gut microbiome can affect the brain's hormones and other signaling mechanisms, reflexes, emotions, and behavior, which you've already seen by how they influence appetite. This has profound implications for a multitude of neuropsychiatric disorders. Knowing this, it's no surprise a wide range of conditions come with intestinal problems—depression, anxiety, ADHD, autism, multiple sclerosis, and even sleep disorders. According to functional psychiatrist and author of *A Mind of Your Own*, Dr. Kelly Brogan, depression may originate from a disrupted gut ecology.[12]

You might be surprised to learn that the vast majority of neurotransmitters are not found in the brain, but in the gut. Ninety-five percent of your serotonin is produced in your digestive tract, so it's no wonder psychotropic medications frequently have gastrointestinal (GI) side effects. Symptoms may arise when your serotonin levels are either too high or too low. High serotonin is associated with irritable bowel syndrome, which afflicts more than 2 million Americans. Low serotonin is more associated with food cravings, weight gain, and depression. Heal your gut, heal your mind.

LEAKY GUT LEADS TO INFLAMMATION AND IMMUNE PROBLEMS

More than 70 percent of your immune defenses are in your gut. Your gut microbes are inseparable from your immune cells and exert tremendous biological influence, informing and directing your immune system's every decision.

Your intestinal wall, or gut lining, is a key point of contact in your immune system. This is where your body encounters most of its foreign material and potentially harmful organisms, and your intestinal wall serves as the barrier. However, a barrier is no good if it has holes in it, and this is what happens with leaky gut syndrome. The intestinal wall is constructed of delicate villi, little protrusions that increase its absorptive

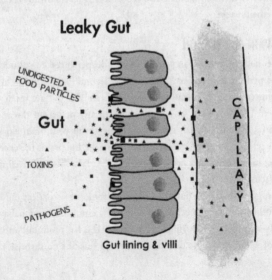

Leaky Gut

UNDIGESTED FOOD PARTICLES

Gut

TOXINS

PATHOGENS

CAPILLARY

Gut lining & villi

surface area—up to twenty-five thousand villi per square inch. Your gut flora continuously instructs your immune cells about who to grant passage to, versus who should be trapped and destroyed.

A malicious microbiome can downright poison your metabolism. If you have dysbiosis, your feedback systems can run amok. The wall of your gut becomes inflamed and begins developing little holes where undigested food particles, pathogenic bacteria, and toxins pass directly into the bloodstream, a condition known as leaky gut (a.k.a. intestinal hyperpermeability). It's bad enough to have crud in your blood, but your immune system doesn't know how to deal with it and cannot distinguish friend from foe, and this lays the groundwork for inflammation, autoimmune reactions, disrupted hormone signals, and food allergies. Your immune system is misdirected to go after foods as if they were a threat, producing antibodies in response, while the *real* threats (pathogens, heavy metals, chemicals, etc.) are given a pass.

Food allergies and sensitivities have become a modern-day epidemic. It's estimated that 15 million Americans now suffer from food allergies, with 5.9 million being children, and the rates just continue to rise.[13] Our gut bacteria play a role in training our immune system about what foods to react to, but there is still so much we don't know.[14] Histamines are key mediators in allergic reactions, and many intestinal microbes produce histamines, including common strains of *Lactobacilli*. This has led scientists to speculate that some allergies may stem from *Lactobacilli* overgrowth in the small intestine, or small intestine bacterial overgrowth (SIBO).

Food sensitivities can cause fluid retention and "false fat," which we discussed in Chapter 3. Histamine and other chemicals cause blood vessels to expand and contract, leaking fluid into adjacent tissues and triggering inflammation and swelling.

THE GLUTEN CONNECTION

Gluten is found in wheat, barley, rye, and a few other grains, and is one of the most heavily consumed proteins on Earth. Gluten is notorious for triggering leaky gut and other problems.

The most serious gluten-related condition is celiac disease. Celiac, which is estimated to affect about 1 percent of the worldwide population, is an autoimmune disorder in which ingestion of gluten results in damage to the small intestine. If you have celiac and continue eating gluten, serious conditions often develop, such as nutritional deficiencies, gallbladder disease, osteoporosis, neurological problems, and many more.

Gluten sensitivity (a.k.a. gluten intolerance) is less severe than celiac disease and has a broad array of symptoms, including leaky gut and increased inflammation. Symptoms range from inflammatory bowel syndrome (IBS) to headaches, brain fog, mood changes, chronic fatigue, and skin problems, to name just a few. Fortunately, individuals with gluten sensitivity usually experience rapid improvement in symptoms on a gluten-free diet.

Even if you don't think you have a sensitivity to gluten, it may be silently degrading the lining of your gut. Gluten is comprised of two compounds, glutenin and gliadin. One study found that gliadin increases intestinal permeability *in all individuals*, including those who have no suspicion of a gluten sensitivity.[15] Gluten can also cause narrowing of the opening to the pancreatic duct, resulting in pancreatitis.

Approximately 60 percent of celiac sufferers have liver, gallbladder, or pancreatic problems. Why? Gluten inhibits cholecystokinin, the hormone secreted by your intestinal mucosa that causes bile release.[16] People with celiac disease show reduced gallbladder emptying in response to meals (low bile ejection rate). Studies show fat accumulates in gallbladder walls, further impeding bile ejection. When people go off gluten, their gallbladder function often returns to normal.

LECTINS TELL FAT CELLS TO STORE MORE FAT

Lectins are proteins plants produce as a defense against predators—a bit like natural pesticides. They are found primarily in legumes and grains but are also present in many fruits, vegetables, nuts, and seeds. We have some defenses against these metabolic saboteurs but they're imperfect, so lectins may throw a spanner into your body's metabolic operations and stall your fat-busting efforts.

According to Dr. Steven Gundry, director of the Center for Restorative Medicine in Palm Springs, lectins make a mess of your cellular communication signals, hijacking insulin receptors throughout the body and instructing fat cells to store that meal as fat. Lectins also starve your muscle cells of energy, which results in loss of lean body mass. The more lectins you consume, the more muscle wasting occurs, causing your body to think it's starving and dial up the hunger hormones. Therefore, lectins are your ticket to decreased lean body mass and increased body fat.[17]

Lectins can also irritate the lining of your digestive tract, especially if it's already damaged to begin with. If you experience gas or bloating after eating beans, lectins are often to blame. Taking supplemental bile salts with the beans may help.

Lectins may also be problematic if you have an unhappy gallbladder. Ordinarily, legumes (beans, peas, lentils) are helpful in lowering cholesterol because they send cholesterol into the bile. However, if your gallbladder is clogged up with sludgy bile, adding more cholesterol to it will only make it thicker and increase your risk for gallstones.

Fermenting your grains significantly reduces their lectin content because bacteria and yeast consume lectins. Organic, non-GMO foods are superior for many reasons, lectins notwithstanding. GMO foods harbor lectins that are new to the human diet, making them particularly problematic.

MORE LEAKY GUT TRIGGERS

The causes of leaky gut don't stop with gluten and lectins. It's common to have multiple food sensitivities at once. Other problematic grains include corn, rice, rye, barley, and oats. The issue is compounded by the fact that grains and other foods often have mold contamination, which is another major allergy trigger (I talk more about mold in Chapter 6). Dairy is a problem for many, as are such additives as sugar, emulsifiers, solvents, nanoparticles, pesticide residues, and GMOs.[18] Unfortunately, most drugs and food additives are approved without the benefit of comprehensive testing—and tests rarely *if ever* include effects on the microbiome.

Studies show that the artificial sweetener sucralose (Splenda) reduces beneficial bacteria in the intestines by 50 percent.[19] Sugar alcohols may be no better. Xylitol is very disruptive to your microbiome, from mouth to colon. Xylitol and other sugar alcohols pass through your digestive tract largely undigested and are unkind to gut flora. They may trigger gas, bloating, or diarrhea, especially in individuals who have digestive disorders such as inflammatory bowel disease (IBD), diverticulitis, Crohn's disease, or gastroesophageal reflux disease (GERD). Symptoms are often dose related. Chronic stress and poor sleep also increase intestinal permeability; your microbiome influences your circadian rhythms and vice versa.[20]

An estimated 80 percent of people with multiple food allergies also have overgrowth of *Candida albicans* (candidiasis). The foods most often craved are those loved by this naturally occurring yeast—sugar and refined carbohydrates. *Candida* produce such toxins as acetaldehyde, and hormonelike substances that interfere with normal hormone signaling, as well as stimulating histamines. Allergies are compounded when you consume foods with high yeast or mold content, like dried fruit, peanuts, bread, beer, and wine.

7 WAYS TO HEAL AND SEAL A LEAKY GUT

Just as a thriving garden requires water, good soil, and regular tending, a healthy microbiome requires tending as well—it doesn't just happen on its own! The following strategies will ensure you are nourishing the good bugs and preventing "pests" from taking over. When your microbiome is properly nourished, your gut will spontaneously heal and seal up all those little holes. In addition to the following recommendations, make sure to address your stress, exercise gently (not too intensely), and optimize your sleep.

If you are having gut issues and need help pinning down the cause, a laboratory test can be instructive.

1. SLASH SUGARS, ALLERGENS, AND TOXIC FOODS

Sugar, especially refined sugars, such as glucose-fructose syrup/high-fructose corn syrup, cause pathogenic microorganisms to flourish. Avoid all refined sugars, artificial sweeteners, and xylitol. Don't go overboard on fruit, especially if you have *Candida* (yeast) overgrowth, as fructose levels quickly add up. Opt for natural sweeteners, such as liquid stevia, pure maple syrup, or coconut sugar, as well as yacón syrup in moderation, which is a natural prebiotic (see prebiotic section, page 156). The sugar alcohol erythritol appears to produce fewer GI problems than the other sugar alcohols but I do not recommend any sugar alcohols.[21]

If you have allergies or food sensitivities, remove the offending foods. If you don't know what those are, you may want to perform an elimination diet. If you have gallbladder issues, the top three offenders are eggs, pork, and onions—and gluten is up there, too. Many people have dairy sensitivities, but some do fine if it's raw and fermented, such as yogurt or kefir. If you have problems with dairy, you may or may not be able to tolerate whey protein. Whey protein isolate contains a very small amount of lactose—less than 1 percent, according to America's Whey Protein Institute. Whole whey protein products may contain more. If you are lactose intolerant, you'll want to test your tolerance with a *small quantity* at first. If you react, then switch to a high-quality non-dairy protein.

Focus your diet on organic produce and healthy proteins and fats. Avoid refined carbohydrates, processed fats, factory-farmed meats, and GMOs. Buy certified organic foods whenever possible, to minimize your chemical exposure.

2. NOURISH THE GOOD BUGS

Repopulating your gut with beneficial bacteria that can outcompete the bad is best done through a combination of probiotic foods and supplements. Naturally fermented foods, such as sauerkraut, kimchi, and beetroot kvass contain active microbes, as well as organic acids to optimize intestinal pH.

Although fermented foods can be extremely beneficial, be careful about getting too caught up in today's fermented food craze. Start slowly. If your digestive tract is very inflamed or your stomach has a shortage of hydrochloric acid (HCl)—which is extremely common—you may run into problems with fermented foods and probiotic supplements. If they make you feel worse instead of better, then you need to first address your stomach acid issue, using the strategies we covered in Chapter 3. Your results will also depend on the quality of the products you use. Always start a new food or treatment slowly to minimize adverse reactions. If you are new to fermented foods, begin with only a teaspoon or two and see how you feel. Increase gradually, as tolerated.

Probiotics can lower cholesterol levels by 20 to 30 percent due to their enhancement of bile flow.[22] Research into the therapeutic use of specific bacterial strains is very exciting but in its early stages. For example, *Bifidobacteria infantis* and *Lactobacillus plantarum* are known to degrade histamines, which is beneficial for countering allergies. Certain strains of *Clostridia* show promise for protecting against intestinal permeability and food allergies.[23]

3. FIBER UP

Fiber is the indigestible part of plant foods. It increases satiety as well as offering tremendous benefits for your digestive tract and flora. Fiber increases bile flow and speeds up gut transit time so that noxious wastes are eliminated quickly from your system. This in turn reduces your risk for cancer and a plethora of other problems. In a 2016 study, mice fed higher-fiber diets developed fewer food allergies.[24] Fiber fuels a radical metabolism by stabilizing blood sugar, improving insulin sensitivity, and promoting fat loss.

Most people consume insufficient amounts of fiber. The average American diet contains about 10 grams per day. Most experts recommend 25 to 40 grams of fiber per day for clean intestines, appetite control, and reduced colon cancer risk. Vegetables, fruits, seeds, grains, and legumes all contribute to your daily fiber intake.

Dietary fiber consists of two types, soluble and insoluble. Soluble fiber dissolves in water to form sticky gums or gels that absorb toxins, bile acids, cholesterol, and other compounds. Soluble fiber slows down carbohydrate absorption, stabilizes blood sugar and insulin, and improves fat digestion. Insoluble fiber helps push matter through the digestive tract quickly.

A specific type of soluble fiber actually feeds our gut bugs—*this is called a prebiotic*. Our gut bacteria ferment these fibers, thereby creating fermentation by-products (butyrate, acetate, propionate, etc.) that have health benefits of their own. Butyrate, for example, helps reduce intestinal permeability. Propionate may reduce asthma.[25] Foods with prebiotic fiber include jicama (yam bean), apples, pears, green bananas, garlic, asparagus, Jerusalem artichokes, dandelion greens, seaweed, tigernuts, and yacón.

4. GET GLUTAMINE TO HEAL THE GUT

Glutamine is an amino acid that, in addition to being a brain food, has healing gastrointestinal effects. Glutamine reduces inflammation, encourages the growth and repair of the intestinal wall, and helps your beneficial bacteria to flourish. This treatment works faster than many other therapies for a multitude of conditions. I have seen firsthand how it heals leaky gut syndrome in just three weeks! For digestive support, I recommend 1,500 to 3,000 mg of glutamine powder daily in divided doses.

Bone broth is naturally rich in glutamine, as well as collagen, proline, glycine, and healthy fats, which can all be very healing to the gastrointestinal tract, which is why bone broth is a core element of the GAPS (gut and psychology syndrome) diet. Make sure you are either making your own broth from organically raised, pastured animals or using a product from a reputable manufacturer *because many bone broth products are contaminated with heavy metals and agricultural chemicals.* (See Chapter 6 for more about this.)

5. LOVE ON LICORICE

Licorice root is a herb that improves stomach acid production and may quiet an angry gut. It works as a natural remedy for GERD, gastric ulcers, nausea, heartburn, and other digestive conditions. One chemical agent in licorice root called glycyrrhizin is not well tolerated by some, in which case you could try deglycyrrhized licorice (DGL). Licorice root is an adaptogen, which means it helps manage stress by supporting your adrenal glands in their production of cortisol.

6. QUELL THE HISTAMINES WITH QUERCETIN

Quercetin strengthens the gut barrier by tightening up protein junctures. As a natural antihistamine, quercetin also stabilizes mast cells and blocks histamine release. Reducing histamine-containing foods may also reduce the severity of allergy symptoms. Histamine-containing foods include fermented foods, aged cheese, dried sausages, citrus fruits, fish, shellfish, avocados, spinach, aubergines, nuts, and cocoa, to name a few.

7. DEFEND WITH D TO PLUG THE LEAKS

Vitamin D deficiency increases your risk for leaky gut. Vitamin D_3 supplementation has been shown to help the gut resist injury. In a study involving Crohn's patients, just 2,000 milligrams of D_3 per day successfully reduced intestinal hyperpermeability.[26]

THE SCOOP ON POOP

Fecal microbiota transplants (FMTs) are gaining popularity and have gathered some compelling early research, particularly in the treatment of *Clostridium difficile* infections. Cure rates are reported at well over 90 percent and as high as 100 percent—no medication even comes close to that! Fecal transplants involve transplanting fecal material from the gut of a healthy individual into the gut of the person who has the microbiome imbalance.[27]

Although this may sound extreme, amazing benefits have been demonstrated for those with ulcerative colitis, IBS, autoimmune problems such as rheumatoid arthritis, leaky gut, and food allergies. Type 2 diabetics have seen enormous improvements with respect to blood sugar and insulin sensitivity.[28] One of the most interesting findings from animal studies is that bile production increases after an obese animal receives a fecal transplant from a lean animal.

Currently in the United States and Canada, FMT has been approved as an "investigational new drug." Some individuals are doing FMT at home. You can find DIY instructions, or locate a donor or practitioner, on the Power of Poop website, www.thepowerofpoop.com.[29]

GO WITH YOUR GUT

Get to know your gut because it's the fountain of all health—everything starts there. Your microbiome exerts a great deal of influence over your hormones and can downright poison your metabolism—which as you know, is governed by hormones. The care and feeding of your microbial army deserves top priority! Eliminating toxins and foods such as gluten, lectins, and GMOs, and cutting way back on sugar, allows your digestive tract to heal and seal, which reverses metabolic mayhem. A gut-friendly diet with an appropriate amount of fiber and probiotic and prebiotic foods will extinguish inflammation, increase insulin sensitivity, and flip your fat-burning switch back to the ON position!

In the next chapter, you will learn how to conquer the final metabolic saboteur: *toxicity*.

6 RADICAL RULE #5: REDUCE YOUR TOXIC LOAD

> All chronic and degenerative diseases are caused by two and only two major problems, toxicity and deficiency.
>
> —Charlotte Gerson

IN THIS CHAPTER, YOU'LL LEARN . . .

- How hormone-disrupting chemicals in everyday products hijack your estrogen receptors, sabotage your energy, and trick your body into storing extra fat
- Why tap water can upset a skinny gut
- Metabolic dangers of heavy metals, such as aluminum, lead, and mercury
- The everyday toxin that may triple your heart attack risk
- How to help your body mop up fat-promoting toxins

Toxins, not just calories, could be dialing down your metabolism. No matter how clean a life you lead, it is impossible to avoid all the poisons in today's polluted world. Especially insidious are the synthetic chemicals that masquerade as our natural hormones but negatively impact our reproduction and metabolism, and invisible marauders, such as mobile phone radiation, that quietly ravage our DNA.

Incredibly, we have *thirty to fifty thousand* more chemicals in our bodies than our grandparents had. Toxins are ubiquitous in our air, water, food (especially refined sugars and grains, bad fats, and genetically modified foods), prescription drugs, and everyday products. Classic offenders include endocrine-disrupting chemicals; heavy metals, such as aluminum, lead, copper, and mercury; biotoxins, such as parasites and mold; and industrial chemicals, such as glyphosate. We can minimize our exposure, *but we can't completely eliminate it.* Only by giving our body additional support will it have the means and wherewithal to purge more of these toxic agents.

Many chemicals in today's world are known as obesogens because they produce estrogen-like effects in the body, including unwanted weight gain. A 2016 study found that it's harder for adults today to maintain the same weight as did adults twenty to thirty years ago, even at the same levels of food consumption and exercise.[1] Why? *More exposure to fattening chemicals and other everyday poisons.*

In a 2005 landmark study, researchers detected an average of two hundred industrial chemicals and pollutants in the umbilical cord blood of American infants—everything from heavy metals to pesticides, flame retardants, BPA, PCBs, and DDT.[2] Toxic chemicals are sewn into the clothing we wear and the blankets in which we swaddle our babies. They're in just about everything we eat, drink, or touch—from drinking water to doorknobs. In 2009, Physicians for Social Responsibility released a special report called "Hazardous Chemicals in Heath Care" that reveals many of the toxic agents you may be exposed to during the course of standard medical treatment.[3]

These sneaky chemicals are so ubiquitous that they've made their way into our water supply because modern water purification methods cannot break them down. For example, even if you don't take birth control pills or hormone replacement therapy, you may be drinking them because prescription drugs have been found in measurable quantities in tap water. A study conducted by the US Geological Survey in 1999–2000 found measurable levels of one or more prescription medications in *80 percent of water samples* taken from streams in thirty US states. The drugs included everything from synthetic hormones and painkillers to heart medications, tranquilizers, and antiseizure drugs. Sampling since then shows the problem is only worsening.[4]

And then there's chlorine, which most consider a benign water disinfection agent. What you may not realize is that chlorine can displace iodine in your thyroid gland. Every cell in your body listens to your thyroid to manage its metabolism. Iodine is critical for thyroid function. When chlorine displaces iodine, an otherwise radical metabolism may turn toxic. Chlorine also combines with other chemicals in water to create dangerous by-products called DBPs, and these are present in most municipal water supplies.

What's the solution? Since we don't live in a bubble, all we can do is minimize our exposure by maximizing our awareness, and give our body extra support. Because it's our cells that do all the work, *real detox must occur at the cellular level.* Your cells must be able to move nutrients in and toxins out to stay clean and healthy. Although detoxification is key to staying slim, it's probably the most neglected and misunderstood aspect of self-care. Real detox requires more than a few days of juicing and the occasional detox sauna. These tools can give you a boost, but true detox must occur *on a daily basis* to prevent toxins from building up in the first place. Once they accumulate, they poison and incapacitate your cells, drive up inflammation, and make a hot mess of your hormones.

EVERYDAY TOXINS AND WHERE THEY HIDE

FOOD		
Heavy metals	Aluminum, lead, nickel, mercury, arsenic, cadmium, and others; copper and iron overload	Fish and seafood, rice products, juices, beer, wine, HFCS and glucose-fructose syrup, cereals, beans, peanut butter, dried fruits, some supplements
Food additives	Nitrates, nitrites, potassium bromate, propyl paraben, BHA, BHT, TBHQ, triacetin, propyl gallate, diacetyl, phosphates, dyes, artificial sweeteners, MSG, sulfur dioxide, GMOs, carrageenan, and more	
Endocrine disrupting chemicals (EDCs)	BPA (bisphenol A), dioxin, phthalates, perchlorate (rocket fuel), fire retardants	
Pesticides	Atrazine, organophosphates, glyphosate, cryolite (in conventionally raised beef, pork, poultry, dairy, eggs; fresh produce)	
Antibiotics	Conventionally raised beef, pork, poultry, dairy, eggs	
Fluoride	Cryolite and soils; teas, bone products, collagen products	
Pathogens (bacteria, parasites, molds & mycotoxins)	Molds common in grains, dried fruits, peanuts, and peanut butter	
WATER		
Agricultural and other chemicals	Fluoride, nitrates, PFCs, perchlorate, chlorine, DBPs, PCBs, dioxins, DDT, HCB, dacthal (DCPA), MtBE	
Radioactivity	Radon, uranium, lead, iodine, cesium, plutonium	
Heavy metals	Aluminum, copper, lead, arsenic	
Pathogens	Bacteria, parasites, viruses	
AIR		
Mold & other pathogens	Bacteria, parasites, viruses, mold spores, dust mites	
Tobacco smoke, paint fumes, gasoline, car exhaust, other	VOCs (volatile organic compounds), pet dander, benzene, perchloroethylene, methylene chloride, dioxin, asbestos, toluene, mercury, cadmium, chromium, lead	

EVERYDAY PRODUCTS

Cosmetics & personal care products	Cosmetics, soap, skin care products, toothpaste	Fluoride, PEGs, heavy metals, formaldehyde, siloxanes, 1,4-D, acrylates, benzophenone, BHT, DEA, coal tar, ethanolamine, phthalates, parabens, fragrance, triclosan, tricarban, SLS, artificial sweeteners, microbeads
	Sunscreens	Oxybenzone, avobenzone, octisalate, octocrylene, homosalate, octinoxate
	Nail polish	Formaldehyde, toluene, dibutyl phthalate (DBP)
	Diaper cream	Boric acid, BHA, talc, propylene glycol, parabens, triclosan
	Deodorants and antiperspirants	Aluminum, parabens, propylene glycol, triclosan, phthalates, fragrances
Mattresses, bedding, carpet, clothing	Flame-retardants, formaldehyde, VOCs (volatile organic compounds), quinolones, aromatic amines, benzothiozoles	
Pharmaceutical & medical supplies	Drugs, vaccines, supplements	Fluoride, mercury, lead, aluminum, arsenic, GMOs, artificial colors, artificial sweeteners and flavors, hydrogenated oils, magnesium stearate, titanium oxide, carrageenan, BHT, cupric sulfate, boric acid, synthetic vitamins
	Medical equipment	Plastics, phthalates such as DEHP, BPA, PVC, PBDEs, dioxins, PFCs, triclosan
	MRI	Gadolinium (heavy metal) in contrast media
Cleaning products	Formaldehyde, 1,4-dioxane, chloroform, quaternary ammonium, benzalkonium chloride, phthalates, sodium borate, chemical fragrances, ammonia, triclosan, chlorine, dioxin	
Lawn & garden products	Pesticides and herbicides including glyphosate (Roundup), 2,4-D, PDBEs, inorganic fertilizers, GMOs, and others	
Kitchen pots and pans, appliances, utensils, packaging	Aluminum, nickel, copper, iron, PFCs (perfluorinated chemicals), PFOA, BPA and plastics, formaldehyde, VOCs (volatile organic compounds), PTFE	

DETOX STARTS WITH STRONG CELL MEMBRANES

Before we get into specific toxins, we need to revisit those all-important cells. Two factors are critical for proper detox: strong cell membranes and good cellular energy. Cell membranes perform vital roles in detoxification; therefore, what you have already learned in this book about building strong cell membranes really applies here.

Detoxing requires energy, and good energy requires mitochondrial function. The mitochondria in your cells make ATP (adenosine triphosphate), which powers the cell. Without good mitochondrial function, you won't have adequate ATP, and without that, poisons build up and inflammation rages out of control. Mitochondrial dysfunction is rampant today, producing an epidemic of chronic pain, fatigue, and brain fog. In fact, many experts believe that mitochondrial dysfunction is the number one biomarker of aging, so anything you can do to improve your mitochondrial function will add to your longevity. The good news is that implementing the strategies we've covered thus far will go a long way toward firing up your body's detoxification pathways—and your mighty mitochondria. What else can you do?

First and foremost, you must reduce and eliminate sources of toxic exposure, which is a primary focus in this chapter and the next. As your awareness increases, you'll gradually reduce your day-to-day load, lowering the stress on your body and freeing up more of its resources for other activities—including healing.

Detox is shared by all your vital organs, so they must be in good working order—including your colon, kidneys, lymphatic system, and of course your liver and gallbladder. As you may recall, your liver filters toxins out of the blood, and then they are sent to the bile and flushed into your colon. Bile is a major vehicle for detox, grabbing and binding toxins for elimination in the stool. Thick, congested bile puts you at a serious detox disadvantage by slowing things down and turning your gallbladder into a toxic waste dump. Your colon is important, too. Nearly every detox program focuses on bowel regularity and for good reason—the bowel is a toxin's last stop on the way out of the body. If your colon is backed up, these poisons remain in contact with your intestinal wall for far too long, increasing your risk of reabsorption. If you have leaky gut, then your blood is absorbing more toxins from your digestive tract in the first place, which increases the strain on all the other organs that have to clean up the mess.

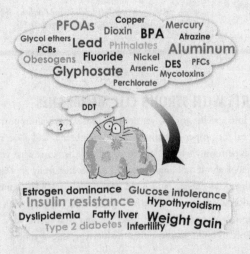

METABOLIC MAYHEM FROM ENDOCRINE-DISRUPTING CHEMICALS

Endocrine-disrupting chemicals (EDCs) play tricks on your body by messing with your hormones. They surround us. Also called xenoestrogens or obesogens, these compounds look just like estrogen to your body and are notorious for causing weight gain. Some EDCs increase the production of certain hormones in the body, while impairing the production of others. Some mimic our natural hormones, whereas others turn one hormone into another. Some EDCs tell cells to die prematurely; others compete with essential nutrients. For example, chlorinated pesticides can slow down thermogenesis, your internal thermostat for burning body fat.

Basically, EDCs are like a wrecking ball for your metabolism that can lead you down the road to insulin resistance, obesity, diabetes, and fatty liver disease. EDC exposure is thought to be a significant factor in the progressive decrease in age of puberty onset for children worldwide.[5] When obesogens target your cells' estrogen receptors, the following can be affected:

- Insulin sensitivity and glucose balance
- Leptin signaling
- Fat storage (increase)
- Appetite (increase)
- Cognitive function
- Fertility
- Mitochondrial energy output

Obesogens are present in tap water, food, prescription drugs, plastics, clothing, and all kinds of other products and their packaging. The biological effects of these chemicals are variable but may present as metabolic syndrome, estrogen dominance, digestive issues, fatigue, low thyroid, allergies and skin problems, low testosterone, chronic *Candida* infections, sexual dysfunction, precocious puberty, and several forms of cancer (endometrial, ovarian, breast, and prostate). The Environmental Working Group (EWG) in the US tags the following chemicals as the "Dirty Dozen Endocrine Disruptors."[6]

1. BPA (canned foods, plastics)
2. Dioxin (processed foods, especially commercial animal products)
3. Atrazine (herbicide often found in tap water)
4. Phthalates (plastics, PVC, fragrances, personal care products)
5. Perchlorate (rocket fuel, also shows up in tap water)

6. Fire retardants (clothing, carpet, upholstery, bedding)
7. Lead
8. Arsenic
9. Mercury
10. Perfluorinated chemicals (PFCs) (non-stick cookware; stain- and water-resistant coatings on clothing, furniture, and carpets)
11. Organophosphate pesticides (non-organic foods)
12. Glycol ethers (cleaning products)

The best way to reduce your exposure to EDCs is to avoid as many plastic products as possible. Read those labels! In the next chapter, we will talk more specifically about how to deplasticize your kitchen.

FLUORIDE AND YOUR THYROID

Although fluoride is not listed in EWG's "Dirty Dozen," *in my humble opinion it should be.* Fluoride can make you pack on the pounds by blocking iodine receptors in your thyroid gland, which shuts down your body's thyroid hormone (thyroxine) production. Like lead, fluoride has no benefit for the body—contrary to what you've been told by water fluoridation proponents. Your thyroid gland can use fluoride to make an "imposter hormone" that triggers weight gain, fatigue, depression, and hair loss. Even more troubling, this hormonal charlatan poses as thyroxine in blood tests, which makes deficiencies almost impossible to detect.

More than fifty human studies and one hundred animal studies now show fluoride's neurotoxicity, which has prompted lawsuits in the US against the Environmental Protection Agency to ban water fluoridation. Besides metabolic mayhem, fluoride toxicity is linked to a wide range of health problems, including bone and brain diseases, diabetes, cancer, digestive problems, and dental and skeletal fluorosis.[7]

Sneaky sources of fluoride include fluoridated water, dental products, processed food and beverages, pharmaceuticals, Teflon pans, and pesticides. Cryolite is a pesticide widely used on grape products—particularly white grapes—so you may get a hefty dose of fluoride by consuming grape juice, wine, or raisins. The risk is reduced by consuming organic produce.[8]

To reduce fluoride exposure, consider installing a reverse osmosis or ceramic purification filter, which will remove fluoride from your water (household filters, such as Brita and Pur, do not). Iodine also helps protect you from fluoride toxicity, so try to include

Myth: All green teas are beneficial to your health and give a boos to your metabolism.

at least one iodine-rich food daily, such as seaweed or dulse. You can also add one to five drops of Lugol's iodine to your daily regimen. Taking at least 3 milligrams of boron daily will also help keep fluoride at bay.

THE TRUTH ABOUT GREEN TEA

Are you drinking green tea for its health and weight-loss benefits? You may not be doing yourself a favor. Drinking too much green tea—or any variety of tea from the *Camellia sinensis* plant, be it green, black, white, oolong, or Pu-er (Chinese black tea)—may damage your health more than support it. This is a classic example of "too much of a good thing."

Despite its established nutritional and metabolic benefits, tea is now widely contaminated with fluoride, heavy metals, and pesticide residues. The reason is that tea plants are "hyperaccumulators," meaning they are very adept at extracting compounds from the soil and concentrating them in their leaves. Unfortunately, this means soaking up contaminants like a sponge. If fluoride shuts down your thyroid, then you're not doing your metabolism any favors by getting a daily infusion in your tea! Instant tea and teas from China and India tend to be the worst, as China is the world's top pesticide user. Japanese teas tend to be better, but since the Fukushima disaster, we must also consider radioactive contamination. Organic tea will have fewer pesticides but may (or may not) have less fluoride.[9]

If tea is "your cuppa tea," then here's a radical suggestion: Swap out your green tea for organic oolong. Why oolong? The metabolism-boosting benefits of oolong tea are well established. Oolong, which is partially fermented prior to firing, is richer in polyphenols and easier on the stomach than green tea, containing many of the same health-enhancing catechins and their derivatives (ECG, EGCG, and the like). Even more remarkably, *oolong has twice the belly-fat-burning capacity of green tea, even preventing your body's future storage of belly fat!* In one study, oolong dialed down the tea-drinkers' hunger by 36 percent for up to 24 hours, lowered their LDL by 29 percent, and increased their energy.[10]

Limit your consumption to two cups per day. Ideally, it would be Japanese-grown oolong as opposed to Chinese, but Japanese oolong is rare and difficult to find. If buying Chinese, be sure it is organic and comes from the highest-quality tea farms. If you know you have thyroid issues, the best choice may be to avoid all teas from the *Camellia sinensis* plant to eliminate any potential for fluoride exposure.

HEAVY METAL WRECKING BALLS

Three of EWG's "Dirty Dozen Endocrine Disruptors" are heavy metals: lead, arsenic, and mercury. Some heavy metals, such as iron and zinc, play important roles in the body, whereas others (aluminum, lead, mercury, arsenic, etc.) have no known health benefits. Today more than ever, our bodies are burdened with toxic metal overload. Our oceans are growing more polluted, with fish and seafood increasingly contaminated with heavy metals, plastics, and radioactive particles.

Evidence is growing that these toxins accumulate in our bodies over time, potentially causing very serious health problems. The effects of chronic heavy metal toxicity are more insidious than from acute poisoning. Although symptoms vary with the type of metal, common complaints of those with a heavy metal load include headaches, weakness, fatigue, muscle pain, joint pain, and constipation. A few of the most common heavy metal exposures are highlighted here—but realize there are many others, and covering all of them is beyond the scope of this book. New concerns are continuously emerging—take the recent controversy over gadolinium and MRIs, for example. It turns out that this heavy metal, known for its use in MRI contrast agents, is not instantly cleared by the body. Just like other heavy metals, gadolinium can be stored in your tissues to cause significant short- and long-term health issues.[11] The list of ingredients and supplements at the end of this chapter will help your body eliminate gadolinium, as well as other toxic metals.

HEAVY METALS AND THEIR SOURCES

Mercury: Fish, dental fillings (amalgams), eye drops and contact lens solutions, nasal sprays and other drugs, non-electric thermometers, batteries, fluorescent light bulbs, paints and art supplies	**Lead:** Old paint, old lead pipes and their water, canned food, food packaging, batteries, cigarette smoke, some toys, and ceramics, solders, PVC, gasoline, auto exhaust	**Aluminum:** Aluminum cookware, baking powder, soy-based infant formula, refined flour, processed cheese, antacids and other medications, dental work, deodorants, cosmetics, pesticides, tap water
Copper: Birth control pills, dental fillings since 1976, copper intrauterine devices, fungicides, and certain foods, copper pipes and their water	**Arsenic:** Treated wood, herbicides, pesticides, coal dust, tobacco smoke, semi-conductors, paints and dyes, soaps, rice and rice-based foods, commercial juices, chicken	**Cadmium:** Black rubber, burned motor oil, secondhand smoke, ceramics, evaporated milk, fertilizers, fungicides, soft drinks
Barium: Medical imaging, paint, decorative glass insecticides, peanuts	**Tin:** Foods, water pipes, rubber, solders, dyes, pigments, bleaching agents, rodent poisons, insecticides, fungicides	**Nickel:** E-cigarettes, tobacco, piercings, cookware, diesel exhaust, foods, batteries, jewelry, dental materials, prostheses, welding materials

Let's start our heavy metal exposure with one that lurks in nearly every kitchen: aluminum.

ALUMINUM AND YOUR BRAIN

Aluminum is present in a vast array of kitchenware from aluminum foil to pots and pans, baking sheets, kettles, measuring cups, and other utensils—you name it. If it's in your kitchen and made of metal, it potentially contains aluminum. The problem is, when your food encounters aluminum, small particles can make their way in and then accumulate over time in your organs, muscles, and tissues. Other common sources include personal care products (especially deodorants and antiperspirants), medications (including antacids, antidiarrheals, and over-the-counter painkillers), dental work, and soy-based infant formula.

Due to its astringent quality, aluminum can irritate the mucous membranes in your gastrointestinal tract and destroy the protein-digestive enzyme pepsin in your stomach. Aluminum also hampers your body's utilization of calcium, magnesium, phosphorous, and vitamin A, increasing your risk for osteoporosis.

The most disturbing implications for aluminum, however, relate to its effects on your brain and nervous system. Aluminum is able to cross the blood–brain barrier. Its toxicity is believed to be associated with neurodegenerative diseases, such as Alzheimer's and Parkinson's. Upon autopsy, this metal is being detected in the brain plaques of people with dementia. According to at least one study, aluminum should be considered a "primary etiological factor in Alzheimer's disease."[12] Symptoms of aluminum toxicity include dry skin and mucous membranes, heartburn, colic, flatulence, ulcers, spasms of the esophagus, appendicitis, constipation, muscle weakness, immune problems, mental confusion and memory loss, among others. You will learn how to aluminum-proof your kitchen in the next chapter.

COPPER OVERLOAD AND ESTROGEN DOMINANCE

Copper imbalance is one of today's best-kept health secrets, and affects about 80 percent of all men, women, and children. Unlike the heavy metals discussed earlier, copper is actually beneficial to your body when present in the right amount. When in balance, copper is responsible for activating more than thirty enzymes. It helps with the formation of myelin nerve sheaths, neurotransmitter synthesis, fertility, and detoxification. Copper is critical for your body to build collagen, so you can't have radiant, wrinkle-free skin without it. *However, when you have an excess, it can really do a number on you!* Copper overload is associated with estrogen dominance, low thyroid, insomnia, fatigue, hyperactivity, compulsive behavior, anxiety, depression, and various hair and skin abnormalities. Copper can contaminate acidic food and destroy vitamin C, and interferes with zinc and boron metabolism. When copper overwhelms zinc, it can exacerbate estrogen dominance.

Just a pinch of copper is enough to make your body happy—about 2 milligrams per day. If you have copper overload, you may want to avoid copper-rich foods, such as nuts, seeds, avocados, grains, shellfish, chocolate, tea, wheat germ bran, and brewer's yeast. Make sure your multivitamin is copper-free. For more information, please refer to my book on this subject, *Why Am I Always So Tired?*

NICKEL AND LEAKY GUT

Nickel is a carcinogenic heavy metal that frequently shows up in toxicity testing, often in high levels in the blood. It is known to cause leaky gut and lactose intolerance. Nickel is also a potential mutagen—it causes chromosomal damage by binding to DNA and nuclear proteins.[13] Nickel is also problematic because it looks like zinc to your body. So, if you are zinc deficient—which is common today—your body will simply grab nickel instead. Zinc plays a role in more than three hundred enzyme reactions, so when nickel steps in to replace it, metabolic chaos ensues. Exposure is also associated with increased risk for lung and nasal cancers.[14]

Besides jewelry, cookware is a major source of nickel, with stainless steel composed of 14 percent nickel. Other sources include tobacco, e-cigarettes (electronic cigarettes), piercings, and vehicle exhaust. E-cigarette vapors are *four times higher in nickel* than is tobacco smoke.[15] Nickel is also the catalyst used industrially to hydrogenate fats—yet another reason that hydrogenated fats, such as vegetable oils, are so problematic in your body. Key components of treatment for nickel toxicity are glutathione (your body's master antioxidant) and correcting zinc deficiency.

THE MENACE CALLED MERCURY

Mercury, a potent neurotoxin, is at the root of innumerable disorders. There is no known "safe" level of mercury exposure.

We are exposed to mercury mainly through fish and seafood, dental amalgams, medications, personal care products, and agricultural chemical residues. Amalgam is a mercury-based dental filling material that's still commonly used today. Amalgam fillings are referred to as "silver fillings," a marketing term attempting to con us into believing they're made of silver, which is only a minor component. In reality, amalgams are between 43 and 54 percent mercury. Studies show that people with at least eight amalgams have more than twice the mercury in their blood as do those without them.[16]

Amalgam accounts for between 240 and 300 tons of mercury entering the market every year. In the United States, dental offices are the second largest user of mercury, and this toxic metal ends up in the environment by one pathway or another. Once in the environment, it converts to an even more toxic form, methylmercury, which is a major source of contamination in our fish and marine ecosystem. More than fifty thousand US lakes now have warnings regarding fish consumption. According to the American Heart Association, men with higher mercury levels are nearly *three times as likely to suffer a heart attack* as men with lower mercury levels.[17]

To minimize mercury exposure, limit your consumption of fish to no more than twice weekly, avoiding larger fish that live longer as they tend to accumulate more mercury and other contaminants over their life span. Choose smaller fish, such as sardines.

If you have "silver" dental fillings, which most of us do, have them replaced with mercury-free composites by a biological/holistic dentist experienced in safe removal. Biological dentists are specially trained in the safe removal of mercury fillings (including the use of dental dams), and some offer adjunctive therapies such as ozone, intravenous vitamin C, and biocompatibility testing.

THE US GOVERNMENT ON MERCURY

Oftentimes, the US Food and Drug Administration (FDA) is dangerously behind on the truth. Dr. Renee Dufault, a former food investigator for the FDA, discovered mercury was contaminating the plumbing systems of many food manufacturing plants, and that same mercury was appearing in many processed foods. When she conveyed these and other disturbing findings to her superiors, she was repeatedly told to stop her investigation, so she took an early retirement from the FDA. In May 2017, she published a book about the insidious contamination of our food, *Unsafe at Any Meal: What the FDA Does Not Want You to Know About the Foods You Eat.*

LEAD AND LOWER IQ

Like mercury, lead is a cumulative toxin that affects multiple body systems, but it's particularly harmful to young children. A child's body is far less efficient at getting rid of lead than is an adult's. According to a publication by Oregon Health Authority, about 99 percent of the amount of lead absorbed into an adult's body will be excreted in the waste within a couple of weeks, whereas a child's body can eliminate only 32 percent.[18] In children, even low levels of lead may cause poor growth, developmental disorders, decreased IQ, behavior problems, and hearing loss. Chronic exposure to low levels of lead has also been shown to cause hypertension and cardiovascular disease.[19]

No level of lead exposure is considered safe. Lead is distributed to your brain, liver, and kidneys, as well as accumulating in your teeth and bones over time. Once stored in the bone, lead will remain there for twenty-five to thirty years. Bone lead is released into the blood during pregnancy and becomes a source of exposure for the developing fetus. Lead also participates in synergistic toxicity with other elements, including mercury, and interferes with calcium and iron metabolism. A deficiency in calcium, iron, or zinc may increase lead uptake.

As you've undoubtedly heard in the news, lead in drinking water from corroded lead pipes is a huge concern today. Your child may be ingesting lead from a drinking fountain at school. Besides being a common contaminant in many imported products, recent testing identified lead as a contaminant in a host of dietary supplements, particularly those with inferior manufacturing standards. Purchasing your supplements from a reputable company with strict sourcing and production standards is money well spent.

Myth: All bone broths are good for you.

HAVE YOU BEEN MIS-LEAD?

Bone broth can be very healing, but you must be careful about the source. High-quality organic bone broth is rich in collagen, minerals, glutamine, and beneficial fats. Collagen is the most abundant of your body's proteins—it's found in your connective tissue, muscles, bone, tendons, blood vessels, and digestive system. Collagen makes up 70 percent of the protein in your skin, so dietary collagen helps prevent wrinkles and sagging. Bone broth can help sooth achy bones and muscles, fight inflammation and infections, and increase energy, in addition to helping heal and seal a leaky gut.

All bone broths are not equal. There are valid concerns about potential contamination in bone broth because lead, fluoride, and industrial chemicals can accumulate in bone, in both humans and animals. The whole idea of bone broth is to gently simmer bones for an extended period of time to create a concentrated, mineral-rich broth. However, your resultant broth will be a concentration of whatever is in the bones. This is a good thing if it's biologically beneficial minerals and collagen, but a *bad* thing if it includes lead or other toxins.

If your broth is made from the bones of factory-farmed animals, fed GMO grains grown with herbicides and pesticides and hormones to "beef them up" faster, then you're not going to want to consume their bones! On the other hand, if your bone broth is made from organic meat or poultry raised on pasture and consuming a natural, biologically appropriate diet, then their bones are likely to be cleaner and more nutritious.

Very little testing has been done about potential contamination of bone broths, so we don't have much to go on except for our common sense. One study in 2013 stirred the pot over toxicity concerns when it found organic chicken bone broths contaminated with lead.[20] Apparently, chickens can store high levels of lead in their body without showing any signs of illness.[21] The bottom line is to be certain about your bone broth's source. Your best bet is to make it yourself using organic bones from local farmers and filtered water. If using a commercial bone broth, select one with organic certification and a stellar reputation.

THE GLYPHOSATE OFFENSIVE

Put on the map by Monsanto as the primary chemical in its weed killer Roundup, glyphosate is now seeping into everything from our food and water to feminine hygiene products, baby formula, and human breast milk. This horrible chemical is scientifically linked to countless health threats. California and the World Health Organization now classify it as a "potential carcinogen"—which is actually quite generous.

Glyphosate's use skyrocketed after 1987, when genetically modified seeds were created to tolerate it, so it could be sprayed throughout the entire growing season. Today, nearly all US-grown corn, soy, and cotton is genetically modified and sprayed with glyphosate.

Many countries have banned glyphosate, having concluded there is no safe level of exposure. However, its use is virtually unregulated in the United States. Ninety-three percent of Americans test positive for glyphosate in their urine, at three to four times the levels found in Europeans.

Glyphosate can damage your body via several different mechanisms. First off, it preferentially kills *Lactobacillus* bacteria, which are an important part of your microbiome. The proteins in your body mistakenly grab onto glyphosate in place of the amino acid glycine, so it gets carried right into your muscles and organs. Glyphosate is an endocrine disruptor and a major metal chelator—so it binds tightly to metals, such as aluminum, and carries them right into your brain.

Glyphosate also makes other chemicals more toxic by blocking certain enzyme pathways in your liver that detoxify all sorts of chemicals. These blocked pathways prevent your liver from converting vitamin D into its active form, contributing to vitamin D deficiency. These important enzymes are also used to make bile acids—so glyphosate is a direct contributor to gallbladder and bile dysfunction. Given all that, it's no wonder glyphosate is linked to so many health issues, including hypothyroidism, depression, cancer, Parkinson's, celiac disease and gluten intolerance, chronic fatigue, colitis, inflammatory bowel disease, multiple sclerosis, liver disease, miscarriage, and many others.[22]

The best way to reduce your glyphosate exposure—as well as your exposure to Monsanto's newest chemical agent dicamba—is to buy organic, non-GMO food products. The key to eliminating glyphosate from your body is found in the process of sulfation, which requires eating sulfur-rich foods (cruciferous vegetables, such as broccoli, cauliflower, kale, etc.; garlic, onions, and leeks; pasture-raised meats and eggs), supplements (MSM, glutathione), and good old sunlight.

ELECTROPOLLUTION AND YOUR BODY'S ELECTROMAGNETIC FIELD

Before you skip this section because you think it isn't that important—*think about this*: Weight gain and many modern-day diseases are linked to physiological disruptions from man-made electromagnetic fields (EMFs), also known as electropollution. Electropollution is colorless, odorless, and invisible—and it's probably enveloping you right now. We humans have as little protection from this kind of pollution as we do from toxic chemicals.

Our bodies evolved under one natural electromagnetic frequency—sunlight. However, we have introduced four artificial EMFs to the world: magnetic, artificial lighting, electrical, and microwave. We are surrounded by microwaves from our mobile phones, routers, smart meters, microwave ovens, and other technology. There is a very narrow range of EMFs to which our brain cells respond favorably, roughly matching the frequencies seen in nature.

Your cell membranes have a limited ability to block these chaotic, unnatural electromagnetic fields, which disrupt hormone communication by increasing the number of receptors on cell membranes. Then it's like an old-fashioned party line—too many people talking, so the wrong messages or garbled messages get through. These frequencies increase oxidative stress in your body, which in turn ruptures cell membranes and damages cellular DNA. This assault triggers your body's stress response, resulting in increased production of the hormones cortisol and adrenaline. Elevated cortisol leads to elevated blood sugar and insulin, mood instability, cravings, loss of muscle mass, and increased abdominal fat.

The bottom line? The more EMFs surrounding you, the harder it will be to lose weight and keep it off.

Man-made EMFs also affect your ability to heal by suppressing your body's natural antioxidant production, including three biggies—glutathione, superoxide dismutase (SOD), and melatonin. A torrent of physiological alterations is triggered that raises your risk for disease. One study found that human cancer cells grow twenty-four times faster when exposed to EMFs and show greatly increased resistance to destruction by the body's defense system.[23]

A similar phenomenon happens with mold, which we will discuss in the next section. According to Dr. Dietrich Klinghardt, an experiment involving mold cultures showed that mold increases biotoxin production six-hundred-fold when exposed to mobile phone radiation. The mold perceives EMFs as an attack, and then retaliates by producing these highly toxic bioweapons. From clinical experience, Dr. Klinghardt believes other human pathogens behave similarly in the presence of EMFs.

It's only getting worse. We now have the ominous specter of 5G, the next-generation wireless technology. It's here *now*, but the fog will be thickening as communications companies release more 5G-compatible phones and other gadgets, automobiles, medical devices, and the like. The "Internet of things" will have us living and eating and breathing radiation like never before. Unlike 4G, plants and even rainwater can absorb the frequencies, so the EMFs will literally rain down on us to be absorbed into our foods.

The risks of EMF exposure are nicely summarized by the late Martin Blank, PhD, EMF expert and associate professor in the Department of Physiology and Cellular Biophysics at Columbia University:[24]

Cells in the body react to EMFs as potentially harmful, just like to other environmental toxins, including heavy metals and toxic chemicals. The DNA in living cells recognizes electromagnetic fields at very low levels of exposure and produces a biochemical stress response. The scientific evidence tells us that our safety standards are inadequate, and that we must protect ourselves from exposure to EMF due to power lines, cell phones and the like, or risk the known consequences. The science is very strong and we should sit up and pay attention.

Obviously, we can't eliminate all EMF exposures, but we can reduce them. Here are a few suggestions:

- Keep your mobile phone at a distance, not on your body; talk on "speaker phone" rather than holding it close to your head.
- Turn off your Wi-Fi at night, and remove electronic devices from your sleep sanctuary.
- Replace compact fluorescent lights and LEDs with traditional light bulbs.
- Replace smart meters with analog meters.
- Unplug and spend more time in nature.
- Utilize protective products that help shield you from EMFs in your personal space, such as EMF protective paint and mobile phone protective devices.
- Surround yourself in shungite. Shungite is the only naturally occurring mineral that has scientifically backed EMF-protective properties. For information, see the 2018 special report "Shungite: The Electropollution Solution."[25]

For more information, check out my book *Zapped*. Electromagnetichealth.org is another excellent resource and a staunch advocate for EMF science and education. Powerwatch has a page on its website devoted to peer-reviewed EMF studies.[26]

BIOLOGICAL HAZARDS: PARASITES, MOLD, AND MYCOTOXINS

As well as chemicals, heavy metals, and electropollution, there are also some biological hazards to be concerned about. Obviously, a multitude of pathogenic microorganisms exist in the world that could potentially make you sick, but there are two biological evildoers that must be called out for their metabolism-wrecking effects: *parasites* and *mold*.

Parasites could be secretly sabotaging your health and weight-loss efforts. Unfortunately, many people dismiss them as a third-world problem, but science says otherwise. One study found that 32 percent of individuals tested positive for parasitic infections, with at least forty-eight US states having fought measurable outbreaks.[27]

It's time this epidemic is brought into focus, as parasites are notorious for triggering weight gain, sugar cravings, anxiety, and sleeplessness.[28] Parasites are among the most immunosuppressive agents on the planet, consuming your precious nutritional resources, producing toxic waste, and eventually ravaging your cells and tissues.

Parasites are particularly toxic to your liver and gallbladder and are known to cause gallstones. Risk factors for parasite exposure include common activities: drinking tap water, eating in restaurants, eating raw or undercooked foods (especially pork or sushi), travel, daycare facilities, and sharing your home with your beloved animal companions.

A parasite infection will send your immune system into overdrive, producing a flood of cytokines that can trigger sugar cravings, weight gain, bloating, constipation, and food sensitivities. Other symptoms include depression, migraines, seizures, allergies, or rashes. Cytokines penetrate the blood–brain barrier and negatively affect your neurotransmitters, such as dopamine and serotonin. If you have these symptoms, it's important you perform an intestinal parasite cleanse. If you want a definitive diagnosis, consider a gastrointestinal analysis. For more information, refer to my 1991 publication *Guess What Came to Dinner? Parasites and Your Health.*

When it comes to stalled weight-loss efforts, molds are another underrecognized culprit. Biotoxins are poisonous substances produced by living organisms,[29] and the most common ones come from mold: mycotoxins. Molds and mycotoxins can create problems in your body from current as well as past exposures, adding to your immune load. Remember, *toxicity is cumulative.* Whenever you increase your body's toxic load, your immune system uses up valuable resources to detoxify and heal. People with weight-loss resistance often have multiple sources of toxicity—mold *and* heavy metals, for example—because their body simply cannot keep up with the heavy toxic burden.

Many mycotoxins attach to mitochondrial DNA to cause genetic damage, as well as damage to your brain and other organs. When your mitochondria become compromised, your energy levels drop and you lose that wonderful thermogenic brown fat. Many mycotoxins are also carcinogens.

Two sources of mold exposure are food and beverages. The most common culprits are alcoholic beverages, corn and other grains (wheat, barley, rye), peanuts, dried fruits, and hard cheeses. Corn is a breeding ground for as many as 22 different fungi due to how it's stored. Cheeses made with yogurt-type cultures (such as *Lactobacillus*) rather than fungi are less problematic for the mold-sensitive. Some of these mycotoxins are endocrine disruptors—ZEA, for example. Zearalenone (ZEA), produced by the microscopic fungus *Fusarium graminearum*, can travel up the food chain into grain-fed meats, eggs, dairy, and even beer. ZEA was identified in the urine of a population of New Jersey nine- and ten-year-old girls who displayed abnormal growth and development. ZEA mycotoxins have even been patented as oral contraceptives because their estrogen binding is so strong—higher than other EDCs, such as BPA and DDT, and less easily broken down by the body.

You can also be exposed to hidden mold growing in your home or workplace. Mold loves to settle into buildings after water damage—and 50 percent of all buildings in the United States are water damaged, including new structures. Mold loves all the building materials used in the USA—cellulose, particleboard, dry wall, etc. It thrives in damp, dark recesses that are hidden from view—inside a wall, under a sink, or behind your washing machine. Sometimes merely eradicating mold can clear up health issues, so it's an important fix. The number one treatment for mold is removing the exposure. I cannot emphasize this enough: *If you're in a moldy home, you need to get out.* If there is mold, consulting a professional remediator is a must.

TESTING FOR TOXINS

Testing for toxicity in the body can be performed by a variety of lab tests, primarily hair analysis and urine testing. Tissue mineral analysis (TMA), which uses hair, is a very convenient way to evaluate your body's mineral levels, including toxic metals. Hair is an especially good barometer for toxic metals because it opens a three-month window into your body's biochemistry. Not only are the hair's overall mineral levels significant, but also the ratios of one mineral to another can provide valuable insights into a number of health conditions. You can read more about this on my blog.[30]

Testing for pathogenic bacteria, fungi, and parasites can be accomplished by collecting saliva and stool samples at home and then mailing them off to a lab.

For mold toxicity, there are several avenues. Tests that go by various acronyms (VIP, MSH, C4a, TGFBeta 1) can be ordered from major labs, but many conventional physicians are unfamiliar with them. If you can't find a mold literate physician near you, there is an online visual test called visual contrast sensitivity (VCS) test, which evaluates how well your eyes distinguish contrast, which has been shown to be an accurate reflection of mold toxicity. Mycotoxins irritate the central nervous system, including the nerves that control how your eyes distinguish shades of gray. The VCS test is available on the website www.survivingmold.com, which was set up by mold toxicity pioneer Dr. Ritchie Shoemaker.

It is essential to make sure you have no mold lurking in your home. If you suspect mold, there is a simple, readily available DIY test called the Environmental Relative Moldiness Index (ERMI), which looks for the DNA of dozens of harmful mold species in ordinary house dust.

EASY WAYS TO REDUCE YOUR DAILY TOXIC EXPOSURE

A comprehensive discussion of detoxification protocols is beyond the scope of this book, but a few deserve special mention.

- **Drink water.** The first may seem obvious but it's still frequently neglected: *Drink plenty of fresh water to stay well hydrated.* A general rule of thumb is to drink 1.5 to 2 litres of water every day. I strongly recommend considering a whole-house water filtration system (see discussion in Chapter 7).

- **Sweat.** Your skin is another detox organ, so sweating through exercise or by taking infrared saunas will support your body's detoxification efforts. I recommend doing infrared saunas once or twice per week, minimum.

- **Improve your sleep.** Sleep is required by your brain's detoxification system, the "glymphatic system," which operates almost exclusively when you're getting your ZZZs.

- **Limit fish consumption.** Unfortunately, in today's toxic world we must start limiting the amount and type of fish we consume. An enormous amount of mercury is generated during coal production, which goes up into the atmosphere and then rains down onto our oceans. I recommend limiting your fish intake primarily to anchovies and sardines, as these small fish have less mercury and other contaminants. Never consume farmed fish. Ideally, purchase your fish and fish oil from companies who utilize third-party testing to ensure they are low in mercury.

- **Invest in an air purifier.** New technology in these residential air filtration systems has revolutionized air purification. High-efficiency carbon and HEPA technology with superior air exchange and germicidal ultraviolet can eliminate bacteria and viruses. Optimal systems remove pollen, fumes, odors, particulates, formaldehyde, gases, and smoke in addition to bacteria, mold, and viruses.

- **Let fresh air in.** Open windows for ten minutes a day to create cross-ventilation—longer after installation of new carpet or paint.

- **Ditch artificial "fresheners."** Lose your carpet fresheners, air fresheners, and chemical cleaners and replace them with non-toxic varieties, such as bicarbonate of soda, vinegar, and pure essential oils.

- **Plants are your friends.** Adopt a few houseplants! Replace lawns with environmentally friendly and bee-friendly gardens, and ditch harsh chemical lawn and garden products.

- **Choose clean personal care and home products.** Avoid deodorants and antiperspirants, and make sure topical skin products are paraben-free. Avoid fragrances (except for pure essential oils). Use natural alternatives to conventional detergents, fabric softeners, and dryer sheets. Skip Styrofoam and polystyrene, and avoid plastics (if you must use one, make sure it is labeled with codes 1, 2, or 5).
- **Wash your hands.** This is especially important after handling thermal paper receipts and money. Avoid "antibacterial cleansers" that contain triclosan and similar chemicals that contribute to today's massive problem of antibiotic resistance. Plain soap is just as effective.
- **Choose clean, organic, unprocessed foods.** Avoid soy, non-organic coffee and tea, canned foods and beverages, and conventionally produced meat, poultry, eggs and dairy. Opt instead for real foods with ingredients you can pronounce!
- **Check out the Environmental Working Group website.** For help finding non-toxic products, EWG[31] is a rich resource for navigating the commercial product maze, with several guides to sustainable food products, non-toxic cleaning supplies, and personal care products, such as cosmetics and sunscreens. They even provide smartphone apps to give you easy access to information while shopping.

RADICAL PRESCRIPTIONS FOR DETOX

If your body is going to keep up with demand, it must detox on a daily basis. Even if you make every effort to eat clean foods and live a pristine life, some exposure is inevitable. The good news is that all the strategies outlined in this book are specifically designed to improve your health down to the cellular level—*and one of the benefits is radical detoxification.* Eating the Radical Metabolism way will tune up those critical detox pathways.

In addition to revamping your diet and lifestyle habits, you can boost detoxification even further with a few select supplements. We can all use a little extra help, right? The following are my favorites to help the body mop up toxins to keep itself squeaky clean.

- **Asparagus:** Asparagus contains glutathione, and therefore supports your overall detoxification. It is also high in vitamin K and fiber, including inulin—a prebiotic to feed those friendly gut microbes. Asparagus is also a natural diuretic.
- **Brazil nuts:** Brazil nuts are rich in selenium, a precursor to glutathione and an antagonist to mercury and arsenic.

- **Brown seaweed/kelp/laminaria extract:** Binds to radioactive particles, heavy metals, and other harmful compounds, speeding their elimination from the body.
- **Chlorella:** This single-celled freshwater alga is able to bind with heavy metals and other toxins. The chlorella cell wall must be "cracked" to effectively absorb toxins. Make sure the chlorella you use is grown in pure, unpolluted water or in a test tube.
- **CoQ10:** Coenzyme Q10 increases the energy-producing capacity of your mitochondria. Ubiquinol is the most bioavailable form of CoQ10.
- **Coriander:** Binds with heavy metals so they can be carried out of the body.
- **Dandelion root:** A very gentle herb that acts on the liver to increase bile production; fabulous roasted and brewed as a tea.
- **Glutathione:** Glutathione is your body's "master antioxidant," opening your body's detox pathways, relieving oxidative stress, and revving up your mitochondria. Liposomal glutathione is a good supplement choice.
- **Iodine:** Iodine is a radical multitasker, helping with thyroid function, detoxification, and combating all infections.
- **Irish moss:** Irish moss grows on rocks near the shores of the Atlantic Ocean and Caribbean Sea. Like other sea vegetables, it is rich in trace minerals including iodine. Irish moss contains algin, a phytonutrient that effectively pulls heavy metals out of your tissues. When soaked and simmered, Irish moss can be used in recipes as a thickener. Its gelatinous quality allows it to grab onto heavy metals and escort them out of the body.
- **PQQ:** Pyrroloquinoline quinone is an enzyme that not only protects your mitochondria from oxidative damage but has been found to actually stimulate the formation of new mitochondria (biogenesis).[32]
- **Silver:** Colloidal silver is an excellent antibacterial, antifungal, antiviral, and antiparasitic agent.
- **Taurine:** A sulfur-rich amino acid used by your liver to produce bile. As you learned in Chapter 4, bile has a massively underappreciated role in detoxification. Taurine is essential for the conjugation and removal of heavy metals, chlorine, aldehydes, petroleum solvents, alcohol, and ammonia.
- **Zeolite:** Zeolite is used for detox of heavy metals, chemicals, and mold. Heavy metals are magnetically attracted to the negatively charged cagelike structure of zeolite, so toxic agents are pulled from the blood and trapped so they can be eliminated by the body.

TOXIC EMOTIONS AND OBESITY

There is no longer any question that our mental and physical health are inextricably linked. Think about how your natural hormone cycles influence your moods! Anyone who has suffered from PMS or the emotional ups and downs of pregnancy is undoubtedly familiar with this. Our emotions affect our bodies at every level—right down to the DNA.

Buried emotions are part of the human condition. Most of us know how stress can trigger food cravings and "comfort eating." However, it turns out that unconscious emotions that quietly smolder over time may have disastrous effects on our health.

There is no more powerful illustration of this than the ACEs study (Adverse Childhood Experiences). ACEs is the largest public health study ever undertaken to examine the connection between childhood stress and illness later in life. It originated in an obesity clinic back in the 1980s, and is still ongoing. The study has uncovered many significant links between common stressful childhood experiences (divorce, loss of a parent, abuse, neglect, and others) and *every major chronic illness*—from heart attacks to autoimmune issues to obesity. More than 60 scientific papers have been published on its findings.***

Emotional "festering" causes stress, which among other things prompts the body to secrete large amounts of cortisol. Cortisol is known to increase insulin resistance, appetite, visceral fat, and weight gain. When insulin resistance develops in the brain, cognitive function—including learning and memory—may decline.

Emotional stress can impact every organ—even your gallbladder. In Chinese medicine, gallbladder problems are believed to stem from one's inability to process his or her feelings, especially "clarifying" them. The mind–body connection is even reflected in the word "gall," which has both medical and metaphysical meanings. Gall can refer to bile, but it can also refer to emotional bitterness or rancor.

The point is that our emotional "stuff" contributes to our physical "stuff," and vice versa. Any uphill health battle may be a red flag that some underlying toxic emotions are getting in the way.

So how do we get them OUT of the way?

---

* JE Stevens, "The Adverse Childhood Experiences Study—the largest, most important public health study you never heard of—began in an obesity clinic," *ACEs Too High*, June 02, 2015, https://aces toohigh.com/2012/10/03/the-adverse-childhood-experiences-study-the-largest-most-important -public-health-study-you-never-heard-of-began-in-an-obesity-clinic/, accessed November 06, 2017.

** "Adverse Childhood Experiences (ACEs)," April 01, 2016, https://www.cdc.gov/violencepre vention/acestudy/index.html, accessed November 06, 2017.

No single strategy works for everyone, but there are some tried and true practices. Things like meditation, mindfulness training, and yoga may be helpful, but one unique tool stands out above the rest for purging old emotional baggage. The technique is called EFT (Emotional Freedom Techniques) and you can learn it on your own. Think of EFT as a quick "emotional cleanse" that harnesses the power of the mind–body connection. It is sometimes referred to as "tapping" because it involves gently tapping your fingers on certain points of the body—some of the same points used in acupuncture. As you tap, you relax and focus on whatever the issue is you're trying to resolve, so that your mind and body are engaged simultaneously.

EFT has been scientifically demonstrated as a safe and effective treatment for anxiety, depression, PTSD, and a myriad of other conditions. It is also an easy way to manage everyday stress, frustrations, and food cravings.*** It clears energetic blocks that keep us stuck—and we all know how STUCK we can feel when it comes to weight loss.

Although many people are successful learning and using EFT on their own, if you have a history of trauma or abuse, I recommend your seeking the assistance of a certified EFT practitioner. For more information, refer to the following resources:

- EFT Universe (www.eftuniverse.com) has a wealth of good information, a free downloadable manual, many training videos, and a page for locating certified practitioners near you
- *The Tapping Solution for Weight Loss and Body Confidence* by Jessica Ortner
- *The Genie in Your Genes: Epigenetic Medicine and the New Biology of Intention* by Dawson Church

---

*** D Church and A Brooks, "The Effect of a Brief EFT (Emotional Freedom Techniques) Self-Intervention on Anxiety, Depression, Pain and Cravings in Healthcare Workers," *Integrative Medicine: A Clinician's Journal*, October/November 2010, 9(5):40–43, https://s3.amazonaws.com/eft-academic-articles/HealthCare.pdf, accessed July 12, 2017.

P Stapleton et al., "Depression Symptoms Improve after Successful Weight Loss with Emotional Freedom Techniques," *ISRN Psychiatry*, 2013; 573532, doi:10.1155/2013/573532, accessed July 12, 2017.

P Stapleton et al., "A Randomised Clinical Trial of a Meridian-Based Intervention for Food Cravings with Six-Month Follow-Up," *Behaviour Change*, May 2011, 28 (1):1–16, doi:10.1375/bech.28.1.1, accessed July 12, 2017.

PART TWO

RADICALLY IMPROVE YOUR METABOLISM IN 25 DAYS

7 DETOX YOUR KITCHEN

> I'd rather have the deadliest serpent in the kitchen than a single aluminum pot or pan.
>
> —Dr. Hazel Parcells

IN THIS CHAPTER, YOU'LL LEARN . . .

- Which cookware is healthiest to support your slimming systems
- The hazards of aluminum foil and aluminum cookware, and what to replace them with
- How to tell whether your cookware contains aluminum
- Are there any safe plastics without fattening chemicals?
- Why you should ditch your microwave and what to replace it with

Before we plunge into the Radical Metabolism plan and recipes, know that the way you go about preparing and storing your food is every bit as important as the food quality itself. Heavy metals, plastics, chemicals, the debilitating effects of microwaves, and numerous other kitchen menaces are just poised to poison your health and weight loss efforts. If you ignore the quality of your cooking equipment, you are raising your risk for big-time contamination. Think about it . . . you have decided to use your precious time and energy toward transforming your health with nutrition. The last thing you need is to unwittingly contaminate your otherwise carefully prepared, oh-so-healthy foods!

So, let's start off from the get-go with some good news: There's a lot of non-reactive, inert cookware on the market today. My all-time favorite is clay. Clay-based ceramics and earthenware are heavy metal-free, without synthetic polymers that can negatively affect taste and food quality. Clay radiates far infrared heat that is actually beneficial to cooking, according to my friend Rebecca Wood, an award-winning chef and health consultant. Wood told me about a full line of freezer-to-oven ceramic pots, pans, and bakeware from the Xtrema company. This healthy cookware line—and others like it—allows for a culinary experience of delicate and delicious flavors.

Many other types of cookware contain heavy metals and toxic chemicals that can leach into your food during cooking or storage. The primary culprits are pots and pans and containers made from aluminum—but poisons may also be lurking in other unexpected places. This is why I decided the kitchen deserved a chapter of its own. Some kitchens need only a modest upgrade, but others scream for radical retooling!

It amazes me that cooking equipment still seems to be a neglected area in the health and functional medicine worlds. Following my Five Radical Rules is a great first step, but if you're still cooking or storing your food in unhealthy pots and pans or wrapping them up in aluminum foil, you can "re-pollute" yourself and undermine your diligent detox efforts. Do you recall what happens to your body with increased toxic load? Those noxious compounds eventually get stuck in your bile and sabotage your best fat-metabolizing and slimming efforts.

As you learned in the last chapter, toxins are ubiquitous in our products today. Often you can't see them, smell them, or taste them—but you *can* eliminate them if you know where to look. Let's start with the most pressing of our toxic concerns: aluminum.

ALUMINUM-PROOF YOUR KITCHEN— STARTING WITH ALUMINUM FOIL

It may seem as though we live in an ultracivilized, totally sanitary environment, but there are in fact some potentially dangerous toxicities common to almost every western kitchen. A *big* one is aluminum. If you don't do anything else, get rid of your aluminum—this is the most important thing to glean from this entire chapter. As you learned in Chapter 6, aluminum can accumulate in your kidneys, brain, and gastrointestinal tract, where it can cause a multitude of problems. Aluminum irritates mucus membranes, destroys pepsin (a key digestive enzyme), and hampers your body's utilization of calcium, magnesium, phosphorous, and vitamin A. It's also well linked to neurodegenerative disorders, such as Alzheimer's disease. *You do not want this in your body!* A good place to start is by banishing aluminum foil from your kitchen.

No food or drink, especially acidic foods, such as tomato-based products, should be cooked, reheated, or covered in aluminum foil. But the risk is not limited to acidic foods. According to a 2006 study, red meat cooked in aluminum foil showed an aluminum increase of 89 to 378 percent; and poultry, 76 to 214 percent. The higher the cooking temperature and the longer the cooking time, the higher the aluminum levels rose.[1]

Instead of foil, use unbleached paper or parchment paper. (You can line aluminum baking sheets or muffin tins with unbleached muffin cups.) Parchment, which is made from wood pulp, is now available in most grocery stores and can be used for baking, poaching, and roasting. It's ideal for vegetables and fish (as New Orleans cooks have known for years) and excellent for retaining flavor because the food cooks in its own juices. There are even parchment cooking bags on the market now. Detoxifying your kitchen is also a good time to replace aluminum-containing baking powders, as well as deodorants and antiperspirants, to reduce your overall exposure.

IS ALUMINUM LURKING IN YOUR COOKWARE?

Aluminum can be in everything from pots and pans to kettles, measuring cups, baking sheets, loaf pans, graters, strainers, and pie tins. It can even be in your tap water because aluminum salts are used in municipal water purification systems. How can you tell if your metal kitchen gear contains aluminum? Here's a trick—grab a magnet and touch it to the item in question. If the magnet sticks, you are basically home free when it comes to aluminum (although you still need to consider whether the item contains nickel). If the magnet doesn't stick, then it most likely contains aluminum. Use this technique to examine your pots and pans and other kitchenware. If your stainless-steel cookware sticks to a magnet and is not pitted from harsh scouring or steel wool, then it's probably Radical Metabolism "kosher." On the other hand, if it doesn't stick or is pitted, it's time for a replacement. What should you replace it with?

HEALTHY REPLACEMENTS: COOKWARE 101

When it comes to replacing cookware, there are many options with pros and cons to all of them. The more we learn, the more we must shift and make different choices based on updated information. The standard recommendation used to be stainless steel for everything, but now we know that even stainless leaches metals into foods to some degree, so we can add this to our ever-expanding roster of myths.

Myth: Heavy metals don't leach into your food when cooking in stainless-steel cookware.

The fact is that you don't really know what's in your stainless-steel cookware. Most is made from metal alloys consisting of a wide variety of metals, such as iron, chromium, molybdenum, nickel, titanium, copper, and vanadium. Titanium cookware probably poses the least health risks in that it's the least reactive, but it does tend to be on the pricier end of the spectrum. That said, despite the leaching factor, a high-grade stainless-steel pan is certainly preferable to cooking in an aluminum pan! Heavy stainless steel is the most stable.

Consider heavy stainless-steel waterless cookware because it retains the most enzymes, vitamins, and minerals in food. Food that is cooked in a vacuum seal without water at 82°C/180°F kills germs, bacteria, and parasites. As my mentor used to say, "This method protects the electromagnetic, healing energies of food."

CAST IRON AND ENAMELED IRON

Cast-iron cookware is very durable, but it leaches iron into your food—and not a good type of iron but a toxic type that your body cannot utilize, so it gets stored in the liver and kidneys. An easy alternative to cast iron is enameled iron such as Le Creuset, Chasseur, or Staub cookware.

THE TRUTH ABOUT NON-STICK PANS

Avoid old Teflon like the plague! Teflon is the DuPont brand name for polytetrafluoroethylene, best known for its use in non-stick coatings in pans and other cookware. In a study published in the *Journal of Dental Research*, researchers found that water boiled in a Teflon non-stick pot contained three times the amount of fluoride when compared with water from the same source boiled in stainless-steel, Pyrex, or aluminum vessels.[2] Until 2012, Teflon contained a carcinogenic chemical called PFOA, which can now be detected in the blood of nearly every single person in the United States, as well as in the umbilical cord blood of newborns.[3] Studies link PFOA with cancer, elevated cholesterol, thyroid disease, and infertility.

If you want a non-stick pan, luckily there are now PFOA-free varieties. And keep your cooking temperatures as low as possible because most coatings are said to begin breaking down and releasing gases after only two to five minutes at temperatures around 240°C/464°F.

OTHER COOKWARE

Glass, ceramic (such as Xtrema), Pyrex, or dairy tin (an old-fashioned baking material) are also options for kitchenware; however, some ceramic, enamel, glass, and Pyrex are manufactured with lead. Baking equipment should be heavy-duty tin or black steel. Avoid brass containers for food storage because they usually contain copper. Avoid copper cookware (lined or unlined) due to the risk for copper overload, and copper pan linings usually contain nickel, which is highly allergenic.

CUTTING-EDGE TOOLS TO SLICE, DICE, MEASURE, AND MIX

Now that your pots and pans have had a makeover, move on to your cutlery, utensils, and small appliances. Start by throwing out all cracked or chipped dishes because nasty bacteria can reside in those cracks. These bacteria will mix with hot beverages or foods and may create digestive problems. Bacteria can also live in the cracks of wooden blocks, so use Lucite cutting boards. Designate one board for meat, fish, and poultry, and a separate one for everything else.

One of your greatest Radical Metabolism kitchen assets is a set of high-quality knives for chopping, paring, slicing, and carving—everything from fruits and veggies to roasts. At the very least, one high-quality 10-cm paring knife and one utility knife or chef's knife will meet most of your needs. Look for knives with thin blades with razor-sharp edges, as well as sturdy, comfortable handles.

Besides good cutlery, instant-read thermometers are extremely handy for testing meat doneness so you'll never eat undercooked or overcooked meat again. For crushing or macerating herbs, garlic, spice rubs, and so on, a mortar and pestle can't be beat. The mortar and pestle crushes the herbs, which in turn releases the oils that contain the herbs' health qualities. The aromas of the ground, dried herbs or spices are nearly four times as strong as the same herbs and spices before grinding. For grinding and crushing seeds, such as anise, fennel, or coriander, a small hand-turned mill is very useful.

The Radical Metabolism plan includes a lot of naturally fermented foods rich in valuable probiotics, and those made in your own kitchen make a wonderful gift to yourself, as well as being a huge money-saver. Making fermented veggies (sauerkraut) requires an extra-large bowl and ideally, a food processor. You can get by with good knives and a mandoline, but it's more labor intensive to slice and dice all those veggies. You can leave the veggies to ferment in glass bowls, ceramic fermentation crocks, or in lidded glass jars. If you really get into it, you can upgrade to anaerobic fermentation jars, such as those from Pickl-It, which work beautifully.

FOOD STORAGE: THINK GLASS, NOT PLASTICS

Food storage is another avenue for contamination. As mentioned, the most scientific way of protecting nutrients when storing food is to vacuum seal the food without water at 82°C/180°F. However, further science is suggesting that all plastics have the potential to leach chemicals into our foods, to some degree or another—even plastic wrap and plastic bags from the produce section. A 2011 study in *Environmental Health Perspectives* found that all these wraps can release estrogen-mimicking chemicals, including plastics with the BPA-free label.[4]

We don't know which chemicals will eventually prove harmful, but we can assume that none is good for us, so it might be prudent to avoid plastics altogether, or to the greatest degree possible. Instead of plastic containers and bags, a better option is to store food in lidded glass jars. I prefer the wide-mouth variety. They are fabulous for freezing homemade bone broths, fermented veggies, soups and stews, dressings, cultured drinks, and nut and seed milks. Glass jars now come in all sizes from little 120-ml minis to 2-litre monstrosities. By the way, if you want to take soup or leftovers with you to work, a wide-mouth Thermos works nicely.

RADICAL SMALL APPLIANCES

As technology has evolved, so have appliances, and there are many to choose from that will transform your kitchen from drab to rad. That said, high-temperature and high-pressure cooking is not recommended. In addition to high heat destroying those fragile omega-6s that are central to healing our body, the mineral and vitamin content and the electromagnetic energies of our foods are lost. Low, moist heat is key. Steaming, poaching, stewing, and slow cooking—especially in earthenware and non-reactive ceramic—are preferable to grilling and barbecuing.

IT'S TIME TO DITCH THE MICROWAVE

While experts disagree and evidence is not entirely conclusive, my view is that microwave ovens should be avoided whenever possible—we simply can't trust them. Our ancestors used fire and put pots above it. While I do not expect anyone to start a bonfire for making supper, I do think the conventional oven, stove top, and toaster oven (mini oven) are more in keeping with traditional ways of cooking and provide a more natural source of heat than radiation.

There are five basic arguments against microwave ovens:

1. Undercooked food
2. Nutrient depletion
3. Molecule deformation
4. Chemical leaching
5. Radiation leakage

According to the World Health Organization (WHO):[5]

Microwave energy does not penetrate well in thicker pieces of food, and may produce uneven cooking. This can lead to a health risk if parts of the food are not heated sufficiently to kill potentially dangerous microorganisms. Because of the potential for uneven distribution of cooking, food heated in a microwave oven should rest for several minutes after cooking to allow the heat to distribute throughout the food.

The unevenness of microwave cooking is not disputed, but what microwaves do to the nutritional value of your food has long been a matter of debate. According to the WHO, food cooked in a microwave oven has the same nutrient value as food cooked in a conventional oven; however, many studies do not support their conclusion, so I'm adding it to our list of myths.

Myth: Foods cooked in a microwave have the same nutrient value as those cooked in conventional ovens.

Microwave heating was shown to distort molecules and induce "protein unfolding" in one study.[6,7] Another study found nuking asparagus resulted in a significant reduction in vitamins, and zapping broccoli rendered 97 percent of the antioxidants useless.[8] Yet another study found more damage to human breast milk by microwaving than by any other method of heating.[9] On top of nutrient destruction, microwaves can cause toxins to leach or "migrate" into your food from the containers they're cooked in, including such chemicals as BPA, benzene, toluene, and xylene, to name just a few.

It's not even completely safe to stand next to an operating microwave! The non-profit independent organization Powerwatch reports that microwave radiation (radio frequency, or RF) leaks from the seal around microwave oven doors, as well as through the glass. Powerwatch says emissions change with normal use and recommends that these ovens be checked at least annually, as regulations are "outdated."[10] Given all the potential risks and evidence to date, there is really no reason to use a microwave oven when so many better options exist.

TOASTER OVENS ARE GREAT MULTITASKERS

The new countertop toaster ovens (mini ovens) make a fabulous microwave replacement. Some varieties do it all—roast, toast, slow cook, warm, reheat, and even convection. These energy-savers eliminate the need to heat up a big oven for small jobs. If you select one whose temperature goes down to 50°C/120°F (most large ovens don't go below 75°C/170°), then you'll have an appliance that also functions as a decent dehydrator for smaller batches of nuts or seeds.

A SLOW COOKER IS A NO-BRAINER

Having a slow cooker is an enormous asset to the Radical Kitchen, making bone broths extremely easy and convenient to make, along with soups, stews, and chili. If you work, your slow cooker can have your dinner ready and waiting when you get home, freeing up your precious evening time for engagement in other activities. How lovely is that? Make sure you choose a larger model—such as 6 litres—so you will have ample room to make large batches of soup or bone broth. Choose one with an intuitive digital interface and a removable ceramic insert that you can just pop into the dishwasher. My favorite is the KitchenAid 6-litre stainless steel slow cooker with the solid glass lid and removable oval ceramic insert.

JUICERS AND BLENDERS

The 4-Day Radical Intensive Cleanse includes two fresh juices daily, which you can choose to incorporate into your 21-Day Radical Reboot, so you'll need either a vegetable juicer or high-powered blender. For fresh juices, a juicer is your best option because filtering out the fiber optimizes flavonoid absorption, which is shown to accelerate weight loss. However, a high-powered blender is extremely versatile for making whole juices, nut and seed milks, smoothies, dressings, and other recipes. In a perfect world, we would all own both a juicer *and* a high-powered blender, but of course you can only do what you can do. The two top brands of high speed blenders are Vitamix and Blendtec, and both are excellent. You can't go wrong with either—it's a matter of personal preference.

ELECTRIC SEED GRINDER

Every Radical Metabolism kitchen would benefit from an electric seed grinder—which is really just a basic coffee grinder. This makes ground flaxseeds super-quick. Ground flaxseeds are a potent source of nourishing omega-3s and fiber-rich lignans, which function as natural hormone balancers.

HANDHELD STICK BLENDER

For whizzing up soups, a handheld stick blender is another must-have kitchen tool. Once you use a stick blender, you'll wonder why you didn't buy one sooner! You just submerge it into your pot of simmering soup and purée away, and you have smooth soup without dirtying up the blender or having to transfer boiling hot soup from one vessel to another. Stick blenders are also great for making creamy hummus, salad dressings, and dips.

HOW TO GRILL SAFELY

Nothing says outdoor fun more than a cookout! However, health-wise, the oxidative reaction of charcoal grilling (a combination of browning and charring) is somewhat toxic. Food can also soak up added chemicals from charcoal briquettes. Therefore, if you're a charcoal fan, please be sure to trim off any charred, burned, or blackened portions of your food. Gas grilling is another option, especially if you have no sensitivity to hydrocarbons, the by-products of gas combustion.

The safest way to protect your food from harmful substances formed during the grilling process is to marinate, marinate—and then marinate some more! Research shows marinades can reduce carcinogen production as much as 99 percent. Non-GMO, gluten-free dark beer makes one of the best marinades! Or, combine about 240ml of avocado oil with 120ml of freshly squeezed lime or lemon juice, and 60ml of apple cider vinegar seasoned with some of your favorite herbs, such as rosemary, oregano, and thyme. For a sweeter marinade, you can add a little liquid stevia or natural sweetener, such as pure maple syrup or monk fruit (lo han) sweetener.

Remember to use extra caution with minced meat, which is more subject to oxidation than whole meat, so cook it as soon as possible.

WHOLE HOUSE WATER FILTRATION SYSTEM

Pure, clean water is your most fundamental biological requirement. With pure tap water going extinct, and with bottled water not always reliable and certainly not environmentally friendly, a home water filter is no longer a luxury but a necessity. Tap water may contain any number of contaminants: fluoride, lead, copper, aluminum, mold, parasites, pesticides, fire retardants, rocket fuel, pharmaceuticals, and an unending toxic mélange of other noxious agents that manage to survive municipal water treatment systems. To solve this problem, you need a comprehensive filtration system that removes pathogens, rust and dirt, chlorine, heavy metals (including lead and copper), pharmaceuticals, pesticides, and other chemicals, such as chloramines and trihalomethanes (THMs). This requires a multistage filtration system using reverse osmosis or a ceramic purification filter.

When camping, do not drink water from streams and lakes because many are contaminated with microorganisms, such as *Giardia lamblia* and *Cryptosporidium*, which can take up residence in your gastrointestinal tract and gallbladder. These single-celled amoeba-like critters can cause chronic diarrhea and a whole host of health problems, including chronic fatigue, irritable bowel, allergies, and malabsorption. Boil all questionable water for at least twenty minutes at a rolling boil.

Choosing the healthiest cookware for your radical lifestyle is both a science and an art. Think of yourself as an alchemist and the kitchen as your laboratory—a laboratory for life. A laboratory must have the right equipment if it is to forge the building blocks of a radical metabolism!

RADICAL KITCHEN CHECKLIST

COOKING AND BAKING

Aluminum-free, PFOA-free pots and pans	Steamer	Stockpot
Aluminum-free baking sheets	Ovenproof baking dishes and casseroles	Ramekins
Pizza stone	Parchment paper	Oven mitts

TOOLS TO SLICE, DICE, MEASURE, MIX, FERMENT, AND STORE

High-quality knives (paring knife, chef's knives, serrated)	Ceramic knife sharpener	Mandoline
Vegetable spiralizer	Chopping boards (one for meat, one for veggies)	Utility knife
Scissors	Measuring spoons	Measuring cups
Wooden spoons	Slotted spoon	Whisks (metal and silicone)
Basting brush	Masher	Grater
Tongs	Spatulas (metal and rubber or silicone)	Mixing bowls (various sizes)
Fermentation crocks	Mortar and pestle	Garlic press
Can opener	Instant-read thermometer	BPA-free ice pop molds
BPA-free ice cube trays	Freezer-proof, airtight glass containers	Grilling accessories (broad-headed jumbo tongs and turner tongs with one-sided spatula)
Citrus zester		

SMALL APPLIANCES

Food processor	High-speed blender (Blendtec or Vitamix)	Juicer
Citrus juicer (easier than bringing out the *big* juicer just for a few lemons)	Smart oven/mini oven	Slow cooker
Handheld stick blender	Seed grinder/mill (handheld)	Spice/coffee grinder (electric)
Thermos cooker	Food dehydrator	Food scale
Slow cooker		

OTHER

Whole-house water filtration system

8 THE 4-DAY RADICAL INTENSIVE CLEANSE

> True health-care reform starts in your kitchen, not in Washington.
>
> —Anonymous

IN THIS CHAPTER, YOU WILL LEARN . . .

- How to detox your bile, flush out toxins, reverse food allergies, and prime your metabolic pump in just four days
- How to give your liver and gallbladder a rest and your digestive tract a jump start on healing
- How juicing harnesses the power of polyphenols to mop up free radicals, boost your mitochondria, and flip on your slimming switch
- All about the forgotten nutritional dynamo called watercress

I had gained about 15 extra pounds while caring for my elderly father the previous year. I had lost several pounds but had been stalled for a couple months before starting the 4-Day Radical Intensive. I loved the 4-Day because it was easy in that there was not much time spent prepping meals. There were just enough satisfying liquids, and I never had a headache from blood sugar swings or felt hungry. I lost 5 pounds in four days—which was awesome because it was a "plateau buster" for me!

—Caroline C., age 63

You can think of this 4-Day Radical Intensive Cleanse as the precursor to the plan, preparing your body to make the most of the 21-Day Radical Reboot. This simple juicing-and-souping detox plan is all about giving your liver and gallbladder a rest and cleansing the bile, while tamping down health-sabotaging free radicals. This primes your body for a metabolic reset.

By the end of the four-day cleanse, your body will have cleared a substantial number of toxins, and your food sensitivity-related symptoms will have faded enough that you will already feel better—and this is just the beginning! You will feel increasingly healthy and energized over the coming weeks as you move through the rest of the program because your body is progressively healing and becoming stronger.

That said, *because this is a cleanse*, some individuals feel worse for a day or two, before feeling better. This is from detoxification, and it means it's working! If you experience detox symptoms (fatigue, malaise, headache, fuzzy thinking, etc.), make sure to stay well hydrated and just hang in there—it will pass. Take it easy and don't overdo your activity during these cleansing days.

As you learned in Radical Rule #2, thick congested bile (a.k.a. toxic bile) is a major metabolic roadblock. Your liver, gallbladder, digestion, and metabolism are all affected when bile becomes toxic. Therefore, a central focus of this 4-Day Radical Intensive Cleanse is on cleansing the bile and giving your liver and gallbladder a rest. Then, the subsequent twenty-one days will thin the bile to get it flowing again, and boost its production, so that your body can easily use the healthy fats you'll be eating!

As a quick refresher, bile performs the following functions:

- Digesting and assimilating fats so that your body can use them, instead of packaging them up as body fat
- Breaking down hormones and metabolic waste, then escorting them out of your body
- Helping you absorb fat-soluble vitamins (A, D, E, and K)
- Reducing inflammation
- Keeping cholesterol levels low
- Playing important roles in thyroid function (and therefore energy), preventing constipation, stabilizing moods—and many more

In addition to your bile and gallbladder makeover, these four days will introduce you to the wonders of juicing and "souping"! These juices and the special watercress soup all pack a powerful polyphenol punch.

Poly who?

THE POWER OF POLYPHENOLS

Polyphenols are important micronutrients with high antioxidant activity that occur naturally in plant foods, such as fresh vegetables, fruits, tea, herbs, spices, nuts, coffee beans, and cacao. More than eight thousand different polyphenols have been identified to date. Antioxidants mop up free radicals in your body, which protects your cells from DNA damage that can result in illness and premature aging.

Polyphenols provide other benefits, too! Recent science has revealed they have substantial effects on mitochondrial processes in the cell, as well as reducing inflammation, stabilizing blood sugar, protecting your heart, and preventing cancer cells from spreading.[1] Polyphenols work together—no single one is better than the rest. The best way to harness their power is to include a wide variety of fresh, whole foods in your diet each day.

JUICING FOR CLEANSING AND WEIGHT LOSS

Fresh juices are part of the Radical Metabolism program for good reason. According to one study, fresh juice was found to amplify weight loss by 500 percent.[2] Why? It's those polyphenols again!

Certain polyphenols called flavonoids feed the "skinny bacteria" in your gut (see Radical Rule #4), not only accelerating weight loss but also helping you keep it off. Flooding your body with flavonoids changes your microbiome in such a way that food cravings disappear and relapse is less likely. In one study, animals given substantial flavonoids showed increased fat burning by 26 percent, and they didn't gain back the weight—*even on a higher calorie diet.*[3]

It doesn't take a huge quantity of fresh produce—less than 1kg per day—to reap the benefits: 450g of produce makes about 240ml of juice. The catch is that it should optimally be *juice* as opposed to whole produce because fiber slows down flavonoid absorption. Ideally, juices should be 90 percent veggie and 10 percent fruit. Adding lemon or lime helps juices stay fresher longer.

Studies show that certain vegetables are particularly good for feeding your fat-burning microbes: those with the two flavonoids *apigenin* and *naringenin*. Apigenin has antioxidant, anti-inflammatory, and antitumor properties. Foods rich in apigenin include parsley, celery, peppermint, basil, chamomile, rosemary, thyme, coriander, and clove. Naringenin helps prevent DNA damage, regulates blood sugar levels, and blocks glucose production in the liver. Naringenin-rich foods include grapefruit, orange, lime, oregano, and mint.

The best times for consuming juice are first thing in the morning and midafternoon when you hit that slump. It's best to make them fresh each time, but if that's not possible, adding lemon or lime will help them stay fresher for longer. If you don't have a juicer, whole juice made in a high-speed blender (such as Vitamix or Blendtec) is your next best option, although not as ideal for flavonoid absorption due to interference by the fiber.

THE WONDERS OF WATERCRESS

What's up with all the watercress? Watercress is kind of the forgotten stepchild of the cruciferous family—a peppery-flavored cousin to cabbage, rocket, and mustard greens. Recent studies have put watercress back on the menu thanks to its powerful health-stimulating benefits, which is why it deserves a starring role in the Radical Metabolism plan.

Besides being a bitter food bile-booster, in a study led by nutritionist Sarah Schenker a small group of women lost an average of 17 pounds/7.7kg in six weeks on a watercress soup diet. The exceptional antioxidants in watercress pump up your energy while exercising, while at the same time protecting you from exertion-related DNA damage, as shown by researchers at Edinburgh Napier University.[4] According to head researcher Dr. Mark Fogarty, watercress contains ten times as many beneficial chemicals as any other fruit or vegetable.

This power-packed leafy green contains impressive amounts of vitamins A and C, manganese, calcium, potassium, chlorophyll, and the carotenoids lutein and zeaxanthin, which shower benefits on your heart and eyes. Thirty grams of watercress gives you a full day's vitamin K. It also provides alpha-lipoic acid, which can lower blood glucose levels, increase insulin sensitivity, and prevent oxidative stress—so it offers wonderful benefits for those with diabetes or metabolic syndrome. Manganese is a critical cofactor for superoxide dismutase (SOD), an important antioxidant enzyme in your body. You might want to have your grilled steak with a side of watercress—its chlorophyll can help block the carcinogenic effects of heterocyclic amines (HCAs) that form when grilling foods at high temperatures.

Bonus: it's a powerful cancer fighter, too. Certain phytonutrients in watercress possess powerful anticancer properties. Watercress is an exceptionally rich source of gluconasturtiin, the precursor of a chemical called PEITC that enhances your body's excretion of carcinogens, which is why watercress shows promise for several forms of cancer, including breast, prostate, and colon.[5] These cancer-fighting chemicals are most potent when watercress is eaten raw.

Watercress is a perennial plant that grows naturally around slow-moving water sources and has been used medicinally for centuries. In fact, around 400 BC, Hippocrates positioned the first hospital on the island of Kos close to a stream so he would have continuous access to fresh watercress for treating his patients!

There is one important caveat. Because watercress is grown in water, it can carry the parasite *Giardia*, so I recommend giving it a simple antiseptic treatment before use. After trimming the stems, rinse the greens and then soak them for about thirty minutes in cool water with a bit of hydrogen peroxide (about 1 tablespoon per litre). Then, rinse the greens in cold water and dry on a paper towel or in a salad spinner. If not used immediately, watercress can be stored in your fridge in a closed container for up to four days.

THE 4-DAY BASICS

During this 4-Day Radical Intensive, you will be removing fat-promoting grains, excess sugar, and processed foods, and replacing them with nutrient-dense liquid foods that go to work immediately, healing and sealing your gut and flooding your cells with nutrients. The plan is very simple. All four days incorporate the following elements:

1. **Watercress:** Nutritious fat-burning vegetable packed with polyphenols, vitamins, and minerals to recharge your cells, thin your bile, feed your flora, and heal your digestive tract.
2. **Lemon juice and peel:** Bitters and acidity to improve bile flow and provide some antiseptic benefits.
3. **Bone broth:** Minerals, collagen, and glutamine for healing the gut, plus some healthy fats to tamp down hunger. Make your own or use a high-quality organic commercial product. Vegetarians and vegans may substitute vegetable broth.
4. **Herbs and spices:** Raise heat production, cool inflammation, and stimulate cleansing and detoxification.
5. **Fresh raw juices:** Low-glycemic, polyphenol-rich juices help your body flush out toxins, build up vitamin stores, deactivate free radicals, and jump-start those fat-burning fires.
6. **Miso:** A fermented bean product, miso is an excellent source of friendly microorganisms (probiotics) to "repopulate" your digestive tract, going right to work boosting your energy and immunity. Make sure your miso is organic. It is traditionally made from soybeans. However, many non-soybean varieties have appeared on the market, including red bean, adzuki bean, chickpea, butter bean—even farro. Just add a little miso to your soup at serving time. (Don't cook it or you'll kill those precious little digestive helpers.)
7. **Herbal teas and oolong tea:** Like adding fertilizer to your garden, these kick up your metabolic and detox processes another notch while keeping you nicely hydrated. Oolong tea is a proven metabolism booster and fat burner.

4-DAY RADICAL INTENSIVE DAILY MEAL PLAN AND RECIPES

Ready for the four-day kickoff?

Here, you will find your daily meal schedule and recipes. Be sure to drink 1.5 to 2 litres of water and herbal tea between meals, such as hibiscus, roasted dandelion root, and oolong. If you drink oolong, limit it to 2 cups per day. If you experience digestive difficulties, consider adding an appropriate supplement. Have fun—and get ready to feel fabulous!

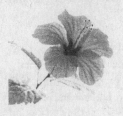

Early Morning
AM Rise and Shine Juice (below)

Breakfast
Creamy Dreamy Watercress Soup (500ml) (page 132)

Lunch
Creamy Dreamy Watercress Soup (500ml) (page 132)

Midafternoon
PM High Five Juice (page 131)

Dinner
Creamy Dreamy Watercress Soup (500ml) (page 132)

AM Rise and Shine Juice
Makes one approximately 240ml serving

½ grapefruit, peeled (see notes)

1 carrot

1 cucumber

¼ head butterhead or romaine lettuce

1 large handful of fresh mint leaves and stems

1 (2.5-cm) piece fresh ginger

1 (5-cm) piece fresh turmeric, or 1 teaspoon ground turmeric (see notes)

1 Radical Lemon Cube (page 199), thawed, or ½ lemon with peel

Clean the fruits and veggies. Process all the ingredients through a juicer or high-powered blender (see notes). Drink immediately for maximum nutritional benefits.

Notes: If you're on medications where grapefruit is contraindicated, you can substitute one whole orange, peeled.

If using a high-powered blender, add enough water for a blendable consistency.

If using powdered turmeric, stir in at end.

PM High Five Juice
Makes one approximately 240-ml serving

100g jicama (yam bean), peeled and chopped
½ cucumber
½ apple, cored to remove seeds, peel intact
3 celery stalks
1 (5-cm) piece fresh ginger
1 Radical Lemon Cube (page 199), thawed, or ½ lemon with peel

Clean the fruits and veggies. Process all the ingredients through a juicer or high-powered blender (see note). Drink immediately for maximum nutritional benefits.

Note: If using a high-powered blender, add enough water for a blendable consistency.

Rise and Shine Juice is great when I first get up to kick myself into gear. High Five is an amazing explosion of flavors in my mouth!

—Suzanne K., age 61

Creamy Dreamy Watercress Soup
Makes 1.5 litres

This soup is not only fat-burning, but filling and flavorful. The recipe makes about one day's worth of soup on the 4-Day Radical Intensive. You can either prepare it daily or cook up four batches in advance—whatever works best with your schedule. If you are unable to find watercress, use rocket instead. If you are unable to find celeriac, cauliflower works just fine.

    1 litre bone broth (see page 216 for homemade)
    ½ bulb celeriac (celery root), (about one 12-cm bulb), brown
        exterior removed (try not to remove too much), roughly
        chopped
    2–3 leeks, cleaned and sliced
    1 daikon radish (mooli), roughly chopped
    1 (5-cm) piece fresh ginger, peeled and chopped
    1–2 teaspoons sea salt, to taste
    1 Radical Lemon Cube (page 199)
    1 large bunch watercress, roughly chopped
    Optional: Add ½–1 teaspoon miso to each warm bowl of soup

Bring the broth to a simmer in a saucepan. Add the celeriac, leeks, daikon, and ginger. Add enough water to the pot to just submerge the vegetables. Simmer for 20 minutes, or until the veggies are tender.

Using a handheld stick blender, blend the soup until creamy. If too thick, you can always add a bit more water. Stir in the salt, lemon cube, and watercress. Simmer for 5 minutes, then blend again with your stick blender.

Serve in a mug or bowl with or without the miso.

Note: If you are vegetarian or vegan, substitute vegetable broth for the bone broth.

I loved the flavors of the juices and the soup! I'm surprised at myself since I'm not a "drink your nutrition" girl. I lost 3 pounds that were stuck on me like glue, so I am very excited about moving forward!

—Bernice Z., age 55

WHAT COMES NEXT?

Now that you've completed the four days, your body is primed and ready for the next phase—the 21-Day Radical Reboot, which is detailed in the next chapter.

You are about to be reintroduced to those all-important essential fats. You will be getting your body "sixed-up" with those awesome omega-6s, of course balanced out with the perfect ratio of omega-3s. You will also be eating high-quality proteins with every meal.

After you've completed the twenty-one days, with only a few minor tweaks you will have an easy "maintenance" plan that you can use for the rest of your life. Your foods list will expand to include other friendly fats, such as coconut oil. So, turn the page to begin building a radical metabolism for life!

9 THE 21-DAY RADICAL REBOOT—AND BEYOND

The food you eat today walks around tomorrow.

—Dr. Hazel Parcells

IN THIS CHAPTER, YOU WILL LEARN . . .

- How to eat to reawaken your metabolism and build a lasting lean and healthy body
- Slimness-sabotaging foods to avoid that throw a glitch into your fat-burning engines
- Fats and proteins that rebuild, rejuvenate, and protect those all-important cell membranes
- Gut-loving elixirs to send your metabolism soaring
- 20 tips for keeping your metabolism radical for life

My first full week is coming to a close tomorrow. During the past week, I have witnessed some dramatic changes in the way I look and feel. First off, I've lost just under 10 pounds in six days. My clothing is beginning to fit more comfortably around my waistline. Hunger is not an issue. I feel satisfied after each meal and continue to enjoy the juices . . . Yum, yum, yum!

—Suzanne K., age 61

My husband and I are feeling really good . . . able to sleep better, and others are noticing that we are slimming down!

—Kimberly L., age 40

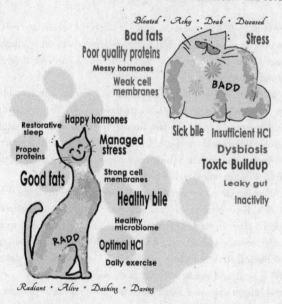

Bleated · Achy · Drab · Diseased

Bad fats
Poor quality proteins
Messy hormones
Weak cell
membranes

Stress

BADD

Sick bile   Insufficient HCl
Dysbiosis
Toxic Buildup
Leaky gut
Inactivity

Restorative
sleep   **Happy hormones**

Proper
proteins   **Managed
stress**

Good fats   Strong cell
membranes

Healthy bile

Healthy
microbiome

RADD   **Optimal HCl**

Daily exercise

Radiant · Alive · Dashing · Daring

Excellent work! You have made it through the 4-Day Radical Intensive Cleanse. Now your body is cleaned out, primed, and ready to begin rebuilding those cell membranes and ramping up the metabolic engines.

In this chapter, we pull everything you learned in the Radical Rules together into a practical, integrated eating plan to optimize your digestion, revitalize your cells, and flush away excess fat and toxins for good. By now you know how your foods can make you or break you—or more specifically, *brake your metabolism*. With the right nutrition, you can turn your body around.

The remaining plan contains two phases:

Phase 1: 21-Day Radical Reboot: These twenty-one days are about learning
how to eat to retrain your metabolism.

Phase 2: Maintenance: With just a few little tweaks, the 21-Day Radical
Reboot is turned into an eating plan for life.

You will be surprised at how little deprivation you feel on the 21-Day Radical Reboot. The cleanse is over and you will be enjoying coffee, chocolate, butter, and cream—I mean, how radical is that? You will be filling your body with raw, unadulterated omega-6s and omega-3s, which is where the healing and metabolic reset begins. However, this is a more radical approach because we will be emphasizing the omega-6s more than the omega-3s, so as to restore and reinforce those critical cell membranes and mitochondria.

Nearly all the other high-fat diets out there load you up with coconut oil, MCT oil, and olive oil—and although these fats have their benefits, they are nearly devoid of those essential bioactive (functional) fats. Instead, our focus will be on saturating your body with essential fatty acids in that ideal 4:1 ratio. Once your EFA reserves are fully loaded, then you move onto the Maintenance phase where you can add back in some of the other friendly fats you love, like coconut oil.

In the following table, you can view these two phases of the Radical Metabolism plan side by side. Refer back to this table any time you need a quick reference. In the remainder of this chapter, we will get into the nitty-gritty with detailed food lists, tips, and product recommendations. In the final section of the book, you will find a menu plan and 50 Radical Recipes to help you translate these dietary principles into delicious, satisfying meals and snacks every day of the week.

If all this information seems overwhelming, have no fear—you can do it! **You don't have to change everything all at once—just do what you can.** Take it one day at a time. Even the little changes will make a big—even radical—difference in your health and how you feel. Remember, this is just a road map. Listen to your body as it is *always* your ultimate guide.

THE RADICAL METABOLISM PLAN

PHASE I 21-DAY RADICAL REBOOT	PHASE II MAINTENANCE PLAN
RADICAL FATS	
1–4 servings per meal and snack, with the goal of eating four times as many omega-6s as omega-3s Focus on omega-6 and omega-3 parent oils (pure, minimally processed, unrefined, unheated) and avoid neutral fats in this phase	1–4 servings per meal and snack, with the goal of eating four times as many omega-6s as omega-3s In addition to the omegas, add back healthy neutral fats, such as coconut oil, MCT oil, olive oil, avocado oil, etc.
BILE SUPPORT SUPPLEMENTS	
MANDATORY: *If you don't have a gallbladder, you must add these to every meal containing fat* RECOMMENDED: *If you do have a gallbladder but you have weight-loss resistance, digestive issues, hypothyroidism, etc.* Choline, taurine, lipase, ox bile; or a combination bile support formula. Tip: Apple cider vinegar or brine from naturally fermented vegetables can be taken 30 minutes before a meal to boost stomach acid.	

PHASE I 21-DAY RADICAL REBOOT	PHASE II MAINTENANCE PLAN

BITTERS

Bitter foods: *Incorporate Bitter foods into every meal and snack*
Metabolixir: *One per day (mid to late afternoon is suggested)*
Digestive bitters: *Use as often as you like; 30 minutes before meals is optimal, or after meals as needed for digestive symptoms.* Digestive bitters and Metabolixirs can be used interchangeably to supercharge your digestion, as well as treating occasional bouts of indigestion

RADICAL PROTEINS

115–170g clean, organic protein in every meal 1–2 servings of non-denatured whey or vegan protein each day Low-mercury wild-caught fish and seafood, up to twice per week, preferably not on the same day Clean animal proteins (organic, grass-pastured, free of hormones and antibiotics), organic bone broths NO eggs or pork	115–170g clean, organic protein in every meal 1–2 servings of non-denatured whey or vegan protein each day Low-mercury wild-caught fish and seafood, up to twice per week, preferably not on the same day Clean animal proteins (organic, grass-pastured, free of hormones and antibiotics), organic bone broths NO pork Eggs can be added, as tolerated

VEGETABLES

At least 5–8 servings per day Fresh, low-starch, high-fiber veggies; organic, locally sourced, pesticide-free, non-GMO NO onions Take care to not overdo leafy greens due to high oxalate levels	At least 5–8 servings per day Fresh, low-starch, high-fiber veggies; organic, locally sourced, pesticide-free, non-GMO Take care to not overdo leafy greens due to high oxalate levels

FRUITS

1 serving per day Low-fructose varieties are best to avoid spiking blood sugar levels	1–3 servings per day Low-fructose varieties are best to avoid spiking blood sugar levels

RADICAL CARBOHYDRATES (STARCHY VEGETABLES, LEGUMES & GRAINS)

1 serving per day Starchy vegetables, legumes, low-lectin grains (millet, white basmati rice, or sorghum) (If you're vegan or vegetarian, up to 2 servings per day of legumes for protein)	1–2 servings per day (weight permitting) Starchy vegetables, legumes, low-lectin grains (millet, white basmati rice, or sorghum) (If you're vegan or vegetarian, up to 3 servings per day of legumes for protein)

DAIRY

1–2 servings per day (if tolerated)
Raw, organic, pasture-raised, full-fat, preferably fermented
Yogurt, kefir, lassi, sour cream, cottage cheese, ricotta, hard cheese, butter, ghee
Many people are casein and lactose intolerant; if this is you, then you'll want to avoid dairy.
Goat's milk products can be substituted for cow's milk.
Tip: *Many dairy-free cheeses (almond-, rice-, and soy-based) contain casein, so be sure to check the label.*

THE RADICAL METABOLISM PLAN

PHASE I 21-DAY RADICAL REBOOT	PHASE II MAINTENANCE PLAN

PROBIOTICS & PREBIOTICS

1–5 servings probiotics daily (start slowly and increase as tolerated)
If you take a probiotic supplement, this counts as 1 serving.
Incorporate prebiotic foods into meals as often as possible.
Fermented vegetables (sauerkraut, kimchi), fermented vegetable brine, raw fermented dairy if you tolerate dairy; miso; miscellaneous prebiotic foods

SUGAR & SPICE & EVERYTHING NICE IN YOUR PANTRY

Gut-friendly low glycemic sweeteners: Stevia, yacón syrup, pure maple syrup, coconut sugar, and monk fruit (lo han)
Metabolism-boosting herbs and spices (cayenne, cinnamon, cumin, ginger, etc.) and sea salt
Health-boosting condiments (apple cider vinegar, umeboshi plum vinegar, coconut aminos, etc.)
Tip: *Reduce dependence on sweet flavors over time while increasing your tolerance of bitter flavors — and even enjoying them eventually!*

BEVERAGES

Drink 1.5–2 litres per day (water plus herbal teas):
Filtered water
Hibiscus and dandelion root herbal teas, to hydrate and enhance weight loss
Organic coffee (1 cup per day) including Citrus Blaster (page 141)
Organic oolong tea to boost metabolism)
Tip: *Avoid drinking with meals to prevent dilution of gastric juices*

READY TO GET SIXY?

One of your primary goals during the 21-Day Radical Reboot is to shore up your body's omega-6 and omega-3 reserves. I like to call it "getting sixy"! There are only four basic differences between the 21-Day Radical Reboot and Maintenance phases:

1. **Allergenic foods:** On the Reboot, you eliminate high-lectin grains, eggs, onions, and pork. On the Maintenance Plan, you can add back eggs and onions, as tolerated. I recommend avoiding pork permanently due to its adverse effects on red blood cells. Gluten grains (which are also high in lectin) are out for good, but some individuals can tolerate certain gluten-free, low-lectin grains in moderation, which we will discuss.

2. **Fats:** On the Reboot, you will focus on omega-6 and omega-3 fats from foods, such as hemp oil, pine nut oil, nuts and seeds, flaxseeds, fish,

grass-pastured dairy, and ghee. Then on Maintenance, you will add back healthy neutral oils (coconut, MCT, avocado, olive, etc.).

3. **Radical carbohydrates:** On the Reboot, you are limited to one radical carb (starchy vegetable, legume, or low-lectin grain) per day, but on Maintenance you're allowed up to two.

4. **Fruits:** On the Reboot, you are limited to one fruit per day, but on Maintenance you're allowed up to three.

FOODS TO AVOID

As you did in the 4-Day Radical Intensive, you will continue avoiding foods that crash your metabolic engine, slow your thyroid, trigger allergies and inflammation, stifle detox, and cause your body to hang on to extra fat. The following foods need to be banished from your kitchen if you want a radical metabolism:

- **Toxic fats:** Eliminating hydrogenated and partly hydrogenated fats, margarine, and overheated oils allow your cell membranes and mitochondria to be strengthened and rebuilt using the right nutritional building blocks.

- **Toxic proteins:** Banishing bad proteins, such as factory-farmed meats, poultry, and fish, reduces your risk for infections, parasitic and otherwise, and lowers your exposure to heavy metals and chemicals, thereby reducing your body's overall toxic load.

- **Gallbladder-related allergens:** Eliminating the top three gallbladder-triggering foods—eggs, pork, and onions—during the 21-Day Reboot reduces inflammation, cleans up the bile, boosts bile production, and heals the gallbladder. If you don't have a gallbladder, still eliminate these foods.

- **Gluten and high-lectin grains:** Avoiding gluten and lectins will improve your insulin sensitivity, tamp down allergic reactions and inflammation, reduce your immune load, and improve the integrity of your intestinal tract lining.

- **GMOs:** Genetically modified foods are nearly always drenched in pesticide residue, as well as being a trigger for a multitude of health problems. GMOs contain lectins that are not natural to the human body. Consume only non-GMO foods. (Products with the "certified organic" seal are non-GMO by definition.)

- **Mold-contaminated foods:** Avoiding peanuts, beer, wine, dried fruit, and most grains will reduce your mold exposure, giving your immune system one less thing to deal with.

- **Teas:** Most true teas from the *Camellia sinensis* plant are contaminated with heavy metals from the soil, such as lead and fluoride. Organic is no guarantee because all tea plants are natural hyperaccumulators. We make an exception for organic oolong tea due to its established metabolic benefits (maximum two cups per day).

- **Processed foods, fast foods, convenience foods, and refined sugar:** Eat out less often to reduce your exposure to bad fats, chemicals, artificial sweeteners, and overall poor-quality foods. Reduce or eliminate all processed/refined sugar in all its many forms (sucrose, fructose, glucose-fructose syrup, high-fructose corn syrup [HFCS], corn sweetener, cane sugar, crystalline fructose, brown rice syrup, and the rest). Even many agave nectars are heat processed to such an extreme that all that remains is a superconcentrated fructose syrup. Shopping around the perimeter of the supermarket will help you avoid the majority of packaged foods.

GETTING DOWN TO THE NITTY-GRITTY

Now that you have the big picture, let's take a closer look at the specific foods in each category that will ignite fat burning and heal your body, right down to each and every one of your 37 trillion cells. Regardless of the food group, always look for products that are organic and non-GMO, sourced from local farms that employ sustainable, Earth-friendly practices. Many local farmers produce their food this way but cannot afford organic certification, so it pays to get to know your local farmers and their practices. Biodynamic farming is even superior to organic.

In each food list, bitter foods are marked with an asterisk (*). Serving sizes are listed for each. If serving size is not specified, you can assume there is no limit. Each food category includes number of portions per day as well as any special product recommendations. Let's start with those radical fats!

"THE 4CS OF RADICAL WEIGHT LOSS"

If you want to make your weight loss REALLY radical, have your coffee infused with citrus with a side of choline and carnitine. You learned a little about carnitine's metabolic effects in Chapter 4, but it turns out that combining caffeine/coffee with carnitine and choline makes a super-synergistic blend of pure radical metabolism power. Performance athletes have used this trick to drop a few pounds before check-ins, with no adverse effects.

It all started with a study published in the *Journal of Nutrition* that discovered a combination of caffeine, carnitine, and choline produced rapid fat loss and bumps in leptin equivalent to mild exercise, without any adverse effects.[1]

How does it work?

The caffeine increases the amount of fat shuttled to your mitochondria for oxidation, and the choline increases fat utilization. Long-chain fatty acids are incompletely oxidized and then excreted in the urine, so you're purging excess fats every time you pee. The end result is that fat virtually melts off your hips, buttocks and thighs! There are no adverse effects, provided you don't overdo the caffeine. You may notice some changes in your urine as a result of the fatty acid excretion, but it's no cause for concern.

The 4Cs of Radical Weight Loss is as easy as one coffee beverage plus one or two supplements:

1. **Citrus Blaster:** Coffee and cacao provide the required dose of caffeine, polyphenols, and other natural compounds like vitamin C.
2. **Carnitine:** Two or three daily doses of L-Carnitine 500mg.
   Choline: Take as instructed on the label, divided into three doses per day. Total choline from all supplements should not exceed 500 mg per meal.

Citrus Blaster (Makes 1 serving)

240ml brewed organic coffee* or roasted dandelion root tea or oolong tea

1 scoop whey protein (vanilla or chocolate)

2 tablespoons cacao powder

2 tablespoons coconut milk

⅛ teaspoon ground ginger

¼ teaspoon ground cinnamon (Ceylon)

½ teaspoon powdered citrus peel (see note)

Pinch of sea salt

Optional: ½ teaspoon coconut sugar or a few drops of liquid stevia

Whisk together all the ingredients in a small bowl, or shake in a lidded jar. Pour into your favorite glass and enjoy!

*If you don't tolerate coffee, you may use roasted dandelion root tea or oolong tea, but realize that coffee is the absolute best for accelerating weight loss. Oolong has 50 to 75 mg of caffeine per cup, whereas coffee averages 180 mg. Dandy tea contains no caffeine. The teas may still work, but coffee is best.

Note: Courtesy of Doc Shillington, you can make your own vitamin C complex loaded with rutin, hesperidin, and bioflavonoids. Here's how: Save your organic orange and lemon peels and cut into strips. Lay them out on a plate for a few days until dry and crisp (or use a food dehydrator). Using a coffee grinder, grind peels into a powder.

RADICAL FATS

Remember Radical Rule #1: Don't be afraid to eat lots of healthy fats! The more you consume (and digest properly), the faster you will halt creeping weight gain, restore your cell membranes, repair your hormones, and create soft, wrinkle-free skin. Radical fats are simply destined to become the most useful staple in everybody's kitchen. They seal in delicate food flavors, keep food hot, and contribute to juiciness, color, and texture, as well as leaving us feeling more satisfied for longer.

One of our foundational players will be hemp seeds, hemp hearts, and hemp oil, due to the almost perfect omega-6 to omega-3 ratio of 3:1. Hemp is rich in GLA (gamma-linolenic acid), LA (linoleic acid), and ALA (alpha-linolenic acid).

SIBERIAN PINE NUT OIL

One of my greatest metabolic and healing finds is pine nut oil. Not to be confused with pine oil, pine nut oil comes from the edible seeds of several species of pine tree—pine nuts. Besides being absolutely delicious, Siberian pine nut oil (from *Pinus sibirica*) is revered for a number of medicinal properties. The oil is about 49 percent linoleic acid and another 17 to 27 percent pinoleic acid. Pinoleic acid is a type of GLA, which may explain the oil's phenomenal appetite suppressant properties. *Pine nut oil was found to curb appetite up to 60 percent for a full four hours due to its effects in boosting cholecystokinin production.*[2]

Because of its stellar omega-6 fatty acid profile and high antioxidant content, Siberian pine nut oil has magical gut-healing properties, offering relief to those suffering from ulcers, gastritis, gastroesophageal reflux disease (GERD), inflammatory bowel syndrome (IBS), and other gastrointestinal problems. The suggested dose for treating GI ailments is 1 teaspoon three times daily, 30 to 60 minutes before meals, plus an optional teaspoon at bedtime. Siberian pine nut oil has also been shown to benefit your lipid profile, platelet aggregation, blood pressure, oxidative stress, and overall cardiovascular health, as well as benefiting your skin and relieving skin ailments.[3] Because of all these wonderful healing and metabolism boosting properties, pine nut oil is used liberally in the Radical Metabolism plan— starting with the 21-Day Reboot.

Raw organic nuts and seeds and their cold-pressed oils are also omega-6 superstars, and have some omega-3s to offer as well. It is best to purchase the sprouted variety because this breaks down the waistline-expanding lectins, and nuts and seeds are loaded with them. As for almonds, unless you get them from Spain, they are either gassed or overly heated, negating all possible nutritional benefits, so be careful on your sources. I have listed spirulina in the fats section due to its rich omega-6 content.

Flaxseed, chia seed, clary sage seed oil, and fish are great sources of omega-3. The plant sources provide the special omega-3 "parent oil," ALA. Clary sage seed oil may be the world's richest source of ALA. Another option is sacha inchi seeds. These omega-3 and protein-rich seeds, also known as Incan peanuts (even though they are not a legume), are an ancient health food native to the Peruvian rainforest. They take a bit of getting used to, but I find that about 30g of sacha inchi seeds is the perfect on-the-go snack, providing an impressive 6 grams of omega-3 fat and 9 grams of protein.

Cooking with oils: Many oils are unstable and quickly convert into toxic fats when heated. As a rule, monounsaturated fats and saturated fats are more stable for cooking than polyunsaturated fats are, but to know for sure you must consider the smoke point of each and keep it *under that temperature*. Of course, processed seed and vegetable oils, corn, and soybean oils should be banished from your pantry altogether.

I recommend the following oils and liquids for cooking. Smoke points are listed next to the oils. Notice that most omega-6 oils have low smoke points and so are unsuitable for cooking. Most chefs recommend heating an oil to 160°C/320°F to sauté.

PREFERRED OILS AND LIQUIDS FOR COOKING:

Bone broths
Ghee (250°C/485°F)
Algae oil

ACCEPTABLE OILS FOR HIGH-HEAT COOKING:

Red palm oil (235°C/455°F)

Tigernut oil (237°C/460°F)

Hazelnut oil (215°C/420°F)

Macadamia nut oil
 (210°C/410°F)

Avocado oil
 (190–245°C/375–475°F)

Coconut oil (175°C/350°F)

Sesame oil (160°C/320°F)

Walnut oil (160°C/320°F)

RADICAL TIP

Freeze bone broth in ice cube trays, then store the broth cubes in the freezer for cooking convenience.

Soaking and roasting nuts and seeds: Soaking nuts and seeds activates live enzymes and neutralizes some of the antinutrient factors, such as lectins and phytic acid, improving bioavailability—meaning, the nutrients are more easily absorbed and utilized by your body. Soaking eliminates about 50 percent of the lectins, but sprouting eliminates nearly all of them. Lectins can trample metabolism, irritate the gut lining, and cause inflammation and digestive symptoms, contributing to leaky gut over time.

After soaking, dehydrate the nuts at a low temperature (as low as your oven goes, 65°C to 75°C/150° to 170°F or lower) in your oven or a food dehydrator. Roasting them at higher temperatures will damage those beneficial fats and create problematic compounds. For example, almonds and hazelnuts contain the amino acid asparagine. Roasting them causes this amino acid to turn into a substance known as acrylamide, which is quite toxic.

Here is an easy way to prepare nuts and seeds: In the evening, combine nuts, filtered water, and sea salt in a large glass bowl (about 1 tablespoon of salt per 1 litre of water). Stir and set in a warm place to rest overnight (7 to 12 hours). Cover with a pot lid. Add a little cayenne pepper to the water if you want an extra kick! In the morning, preheat your oven to 65°C/150°F (or use a food dehydrator). Rinse the nuts and seeds in a colander, and then spread them onto a baking sheet in a single layer. Leave in the oven for 6 to 24 hours, giving an occasional stir. Allow to cool completely before storing.

Storage: Keep your oils, nuts, and seeds in the refrigerator or freezer. Here's a tip: For extra insurance that your oils will stay fresh, add one drop of vitamin E oil from a capsule right into the bottle of oil!

Servings per day on Reboot and Maintenance: One to four servings per day, with four times as many omega-6s as omega-3s (as close as you can to achieve that 4:1 ratio).

RADICAL FATS

Fats are listed by category. The term *neutral* refers to fats that do not affect your omega-6 to omega-3 ratio. Temperatures in parentheses represent smoke points.

OMEGA-6 FATS

Almonds and almond oil (215°C/420°F), 1 tablespoon oil or 7 almonds

Hazelnuts and hazelnut oil (215°C/420°F), 1 tablespoon or 6 hazelnuts

*Hemp seeds, hemp hearts, and hemp oil (165°C/325°F), 1 tablespoon

*Sesame seeds, sesame oil, tahini (160°C/320°F), 1 tablespoon

Walnuts, walnut oil, walnut butter (160°C/320°F), 1 tablespoon or 4 walnut halves

Sunflower seeds, oil, butter (105°C/225°F), 1 tablespoon

High-linoleic safflower oil (105°C/225°F), 1 tablespoon

Pine nuts, pine nut oil, 1 tablespoon oil or 2 tablespoons pine nuts

*Apricot kernels and apricot kernel oil, 1 tablespoon oil or 3 kernels

*Black seed oil, 1 teaspoon

Pumpkin seeds and oil, pumpkin seed butter, 1 tablespoon

Pecans and pecan butter, 1 tablespoon

Cashews and cashew butter, 1 tablespoon butter or 6 cashews

Pistachios, 15 nuts

Brazil nuts, 2 medium-size

Pastured butter (165°C/330°F), 1 tablespoon

Ghee (250°C/485°F), 1 tablespoon

Pastured cream, 1 tablespoon

Spirulina, 2 tablespoons

OMEGA-3 FATS

Flaxseed and high-lignan flaxseed oil (105°C/225°F), 1 tablespoon oil or 3 tablespoons ground toasted flaxseed

Chia seed, 1 tablespoon

Perilla seed oil, 1 teaspoon

Clary sage seed oil, 1 teaspoon

Sacha inchi seeds/Incan peanuts, 30g

Fish or fish oil, 1 tablespoon

NEUTRAL OILS

Tigernut oil (237°C/460°F), 1 tablespoon

Palm oil (235°C/455°F), 1

tablespoon (only products certified by the Roundtable on Sustainable Palm Oil, an organization that supports growers who use minimal pesticides and don't clear-cut rainforests)

Macadamia nuts and oil (210°C/410°F), 3 nuts or 1 tablespoon oil

Algae oil, 1 teaspoon

Beef tallow (dripping) (205°C/400°F), 1 tablespoon

Avocado oil (virgin) (190–245°C/375–475°F), 1 tablespoon

Chicken fat (190°C/375°F), 1 tablespoon

Duck or goose fat

(190°C/375°F), 1 tablespoon

Lard (185°C/370°F), 1 tablespoon

Coconut, coconut cream, coconut oil (175°C/350°F for coconut oil), 1 tablespoon coconut cream or 2 tablespoons shredded coconut

Extra-virgin olive oil (105–160°C/220–320°F), 1 tablespoon

Coconut milk, 6 tablespoons (90ml)

MCT oil, 1 tablespoon

*Uncured olives, 8 olives

BITTERS

As you learned in the gallbladder chapter, bitters get our digestive juices flowing by

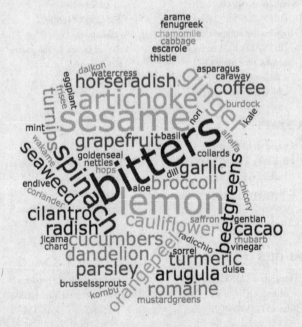

stimulating the release of saliva, hydrochloric acid (HCl), bile, pepsin, gastrin and pancreatic enzymes, as well as increasing lower esophageal sphincter (LES) tone. There are three ways to get your bitters:

1. **Bitter foods:** Introduce more bitter foods directly into your diet every day. See table on page 53.
2. **Digestive bitters:** Concentrated, bitter plant-based tinctures to take before a meal, after a meal, or any time you experience digestive symptoms. There are several excellent digestive bitters on the market.
3. **Metabolixirs:** I have developed three bitter aperitifs called "Metabolixirs." These kick the digestive bitters up another notch—they have digestive bitters as one ingredient, but they supercharge your digestion and metabolism even more with a few key ingredients, such as apple cider vinegar and thermogenic herbs and spices.

During the 21-Day Radical Reboot, you will be reacquainting yourself with bitter foods by including at least one with every meal and snack. But we won't stop there—you will boost your bitters further with the addition of an afternoon Metabolixir. These do everything digestive bitters do, *and then some.* The Metabolixirs do not replace bitter foods in your meals—they add to them.

THE AMAZING METABOLIXIRS

The afternoon Metabolixir replaces the afternoon juice you were consuming on the 4-Day Intensive Cleanse. However, if you don't want to let that juice go, then it's completely fine to have both.

The Metabolixirs boost stomach acid, increase digestive juices, stimulate bile flow, and help relieve indigestion or GERD. They have additional herbs to flip on your metabolic afterburners. If you're on the go or rushed, no worries—just do a squirt of the plain bitters instead. I want you to have plenty of options.

There are three Metabolixir recipes to choose from (pages 196–197). Feel free to modify them and make them your own, and mix and match to your heart's content. For example, you can have one thirty minutes before each meal, and between meals, as well as after a meal if you experience indigestion. Metabolixirs are a great way to get your bitters *and* apple cider vinegar down in one gulp.

Servings: Incorporate bitter foods into every meal and snack; *plus*, add one Metabolixir in the mid- to late afternoon (replaces the second juice you were consuming on the 4-Day Intensive Cleanse); you can also add a dose of digestive bitters as often as you like—thirty minutes before meals is optimal, but they may also be helpful after meals as needed for indigestion.

For a complete list of bitter foods, refer back to the table on page 53.

RADICAL TIPS: BITTERS

A shot glass or jigger is handy for mixing the Metabolixirs.

Sauerkraut brine is an alternative digestif.

Mountain Rose Herbs has a simple recipe for making your own digestive bitters from dandelion root, fennel seeds, ginger, and orange peel.[4]

RADICAL PROTEINS

Radical proteins will supply much-needed amino acids for activating muscle tissue and firing up your mitochondria. Make sure your meats are organically raised on pasture. Conventionally raised meats may be loaded with chemicals, growth-stimulating hormones, antibiotics, GMOs, and harmful plant lectins from the corn and soy in their feed.

Myth: All soy products are bad for you.

Aim for 20 grams of protein with each meal, which is roughly 115–170g of meat or poultry. Add one or two servings of whey protein per day. If you're vegan, substitute tempeh for the animal proteins, and rice and pea protein powder for the whey. Why tempeh? Tempeh is the healthy soy.

Move over tofu—you've been replaced! Unlike tofu, tempeh is a *fermented* soybean product, so it has none of the problematic issues of tofu. Besides that, it has some impressive health benefits. First of all, because it's fermented, tempeh is a probiotic food. It has also been shown to reduce cholesterol and LDL levels. Tempeh's isoflavones have benefits for menopausal symptoms, including easing hot flashes. It lowers circulating estrogen levels and acts as an adaptogen, not to mention having anticancer and anti-inflammatory benefits.

During the Reboot, you'll be eliminating the top allergens associated with gallbladder problems, which include pork and eggs—with eggs being number one. Although you can add eggs back to your diet on Maintenance, I recommend avoiding pork permanently because it tends to cause extreme red blood cell clumping (hypercoagulation).[5] Bitters and HCl replacements, such as apple cider vinegar, will help you extract those valuable aminos from your proteins. You can also supplement your protein intake with an MAP supplement.

Servings per day on Reboot: 115–170g of protein in every meal (no pork or eggs), plus 1 to 2 servings of non-denatured whey or vegan protein each day. Limit fish and seafood to twice per week, preferably not on same day.

Servings per day on Maintenance: 115–170g of protein in every meal (no pork; eggs only if tolerated), plus 1 to 2 servings of nondenatured whey or vegan protein each day. Limit fish and seafood to twice per week, preferably not on the same day.

RADICAL PROTEINS

Grass-pastured beef
Grass-pastured bison and buffalo
Grass-pastured lamb
Grass-pastured poultry
Organic bone broths
Low-mercury tuna
Wild-caught salmon
Sardines

Seafood, e.g. prawns, scallops, lobster, oysters, mussels, crab
Anchovies
Oysters
Mackerel
Hempfu (hemp tofu)
Tempeh
Whey protein,

undenatured and unheated from grass-fed A2 cows
Vegan pea and rice protein powder
Hempseed powder
Spirulina

VEGETABLES

Vegetables are the staff of life—*not grains!* Veggies should be part of every meal and snack, as well as representing the majority of what goes into your fresh raw juices. There are only a few cautions when it comes to veggies.

Onions are avoided while on the Reboot because of their association with gall-bladder problems. You can gradually add them back in on Maintenance—as always, carefully monitor how you feel. Despite their nutritional benefits, mushrooms are best avoided altogether due to common mycotoxin sensitivities.

Nightshades (tomatoes, white potatoes, aubergines, peppers and chili peppers, tomatillos, etc.) are avoided by many due to their association with joint pain, inflammation, and autoimmune issues, such as rheumatoid arthritis (RA), possibly related to their alkaloid and lectin content. People with a compromised gut often have problems with nightshades, so to optimize your gut healing it's wise to avoid them, at least for a while. The exceptions are spices derived from nightshades (cayenne pepper, paprika, red pepper flakes), which I've rarely seen cause a problem. If you are nightshade sensitive, just be mindful.

Some folks are sensitive to naturally occurring compounds called oxalates, which are found in a wide variety of vegetables and other foods. They are sometimes not metabolized properly, especially when you consume more than your system can handle. Oxalate buildup can interfere with gallbladder function, digestion, detoxification, and important metabolic processes.[6] Oxalate levels vary with type and source but are highest in rhubarb, spinach, beet greens, Swiss chard, and other leafy greens; cacao; berries; cashews; peanuts and other legumes; and grains. Oxalates are also commonly found in processed foods. Admittedly, oxalates can be found in many Radical Metabolism foods and it's impossible to eliminate all of them, but if you know you are sensitive, then it's wise to take precautions. Leafy greens, such as spinach, have some of the highest oxalate, so individuals regularly consuming green juices or smoothies may be getting too many oxalates if they're juicing a lot of greens. Oh my—it looks like we just busted another myth.

> Myth: You can't eat too many leafy green vegetables.

Now you know why you actually can *eat too many leafy greens!* Don't get me wrong, greens are good, but if, in your efforts to improve your health you've morphed into a greens addict, back off a bit from the spinach and chard. Kale is an exception, being relatively low in oxalates. Replace them with some of the other fabulous veggies that are lower in oxalates—celery, cucumbers, green beans, courgettes, and jicama (yam beans). Variety is the spice of life!

RADICAL TIPS: VEGGIES

- **Peeling and seeding:** Peel and remove the seeds from such vegetables as aubergines, peppers, tomatoes, cucumbers, summer squash, and winter squash to remove lectins. An easy way to peel tomatoes is to drop them into boiling water for 60 seconds, or roast them under a grill for 15 minutes. When they are cool, the skins slide off easily. Peppers can also be roasted and peeled, or skinned with a peeler. To remove

the seeds from a tomato, cut it in half around its equator, and then scoop out the seeds and pith from the seed cavities in each half.

- **Veggies in the fridge:** If you have readily accessible prepped veggies in the front of your fridge, you are less likely to stray from your plan. Keep asparagus, cucumber, carrot, and celery sticks fresh and crisp by storing them in a covered glass jar with a bit of water—at easy arm's reach!

- **Veggies in the freezer:** Keep a stash of veggies in your freezer. Good candidates are asparagus, kale, spinach, peas, broccoli, green beans, squash, artichoke hearts, and okra.

- **Veggies in the pantry**: Stock your pantry with basic veggie staples preserved in cans or glass: artichoke hearts, bamboo shoots, hearts of palm, water chestnuts.

Servings: At least 5 to 8 servings per day (not including juice).

Reminder: Go for those bitters! Bitters are flagged with an asterisk (*). There are many to choose from in the land of vegetables.

VEGETABLES

*Alfalfa sprouts	*Dandelion greens	*Rapini (cime di rapa)
*Artichokes	*Endive	*Romaine lettuce
*Arugula (rocket)	*Escarole	*Red leaf lettuce
*Asparagus	*Frisée	*Rhubarb
*Beet greens	Green beans	*Spring greens
Bamboo shoots	Hearts of palm	Spring onions
*Broccoli	*Jerusalem artichoke	Shallots
*Brussels sprouts	*Jicama (yam beans)	*Spinach
*Burdock	*Kale	Squash (spaghetti,
*Cabbage	Leafy greens	summer, courgettes)
*Cauliflower	Leeks	*Swiss chard
Celery	Lemon grass	*Turnip greens
*Chicory	*Mustard greens	Water chestnuts
*Chilies	*Nettles	*Watercress
Chives	*Pumpkin	*Wild lettuce
*Cucumber	*Radicchio	
*Daikon radish (mooli)	*Radish	

FRUITS

Fruits are loaded with wonderful vitamins, minerals, antioxidants, fiber, and other essential nutrients, but they can also be high in natural sugar (fructose), so it's possible to overdo them. Fruits lowest in fructose are berries, kiwis, lemons, limes, and avocados (Maintenance), which of course are bursting with beneficial fats. These low-sugar fruits contain excellent nutrients—did you know a single kiwi fruit has *twice the vitamin C* of an orange? Fruits should be eaten alone unless blended into a smoothie. Dried fruits are problematic because of mold contamination, as well as how easy they are to overconsume.

Servings on Reboot: 1 serving per day (not including juices).
Servings on Maintenance: 1 to 3 servings per day (not including juices).
*Reminder: Don't forget to include those bitters!

FRUITS

Apple (1 small)
Apricots (2 medium)
Avocado (½ small)
Banana (½ small)
Berries (seasonal) (70g)
*Bitter melon
Cherries (10)
Grapes (12)
*Grapefruit (½)
Kiwi (1 medium)

*Lemon (including peel/rind)
* Lime (including peel/rind)
Mango (80g)
Melon (honeydew, cantaloupe, watermelon, others) (⅛; 150g watermelon)
Nectarine (1 small)
Orange (1 small)

*Orange peel/rind
Papaya (½)
Peach (1 medium)
Pear (1 small)
Pineapple (80g)
Plums (2 medium)
Pomegranate (1)
Tangerine (1 large)
*Tangerine peel/rind

RADICAL CARBOHYDRATES (STARCHY VEGETABLES, LEGUMES & GRAINS)

Starches are our "comfort foods" and are allowed in moderation. They also provide fiber and fullness. Starchy vegetables and legumes are the safest sources. Grains can be problematic for several reasons, including gluten issues, lectins, pesticide residues, and mold contamination. There are no nutrients in grains that are not obtainable from other foods. The United States has the world's worst mold contamination problem, and grains are especially notorious. They are also notorious for causing insulin resistance and stalling weight loss. I suggest avoiding *all* glutenous grains and, depending on your sensitivity, you might decide to go grain-free for life—which I commend!

During both Reboot and Maintenance, we eliminate all grains except for three that are very low in lectins: millet, sorghum, and white basmati rice. While you might still choose to avoid *all* grains, some individuals are able to tolerate low-lectin grains, which is why these three are the best options. Why not quinoa? Although quinoa is gluten-free and relatively high in protein, you also get a hefty dose of weight-loss-stalling lectins.

Just keep this in mind: If you are not getting the results you want from the plan or you continue to experience digestive issues, grains would be the first thing to eliminate.

Gluten: Besides being highly problematic for people with celiac disease, gluten may cause inflammation, insulin resistance, and intestinal damage, even if you aren't celiac, at least for those who are sensitive—*and this appears to be a majority of us.* Many people are gluten sensitive without realizing it.

Lectins: Abundant in many grains and legumes (plus other foods), lectins throw a wrench into your metabolic operations so are best minimized. Lectins can stall fat burning by making a mess of cellular communication and stimulating appetite and fat storage. Lectins can also irritate the lining of your digestive tract, leading to gas and bloating.

Phytic acid: Grains produce phytic acid as a defense against foragers. When consumed, phytic acid binds to minerals and prevents their absorption. If consumed often enough, mineral deficiencies can develop.

Peanuts: Peanuts are omitted from the plan for one reason only: they are highly susceptible to mold—even organic varieties. I'm the first person to protest this omission—I feel your pain. *I'm totally nuts about peanuts!* However, mold sensitivities are such a huge issue that I cannot in good conscience allow them in the plan, or in my kitchen.

RADICAL TIPS: CARBS

Soak 'em: Some of the problematic effects of grains, legumes, nuts, and seeds can be lessened by soaking or sprouting.

For beans, run them through a "presoak cycle": Soak for at least 12 hours before cooking, and add apple cider vinegar to the water. The addition of bicarbonate of soda is said to boost lectin neutralization. After soaking, rinse well and use fresh water for cooking. Cooking for at least 15 minutes on high heat is said to reduce lectin toxicity by 500 percent. Alternatively, both lectins and phytic acids can be destroyed by cooking beans in a pressure cooker. Slow cookers actually *increase* lectin content. As a work-around, finish off your slow-cooker beans with a 15-minute blast of high heat on the stove top.

Do you miss noodles? "Miracle noodles" (shirataki, a.k.a. white waterfall noodles) are a calorie-free, starch-free noodle made from high-fiber konjac glucomannan, from the Asian yam family. Glucomannan is also a prebiotic. You can add these noodles to soups, stir-fries, or other dishes with reckless abandon because they are essentially calorie-free.

Servings on Reboot: 1 complex carb serving per day; vegans or vegetarians are allowed up to 2 servings of legumes per day because they serve as a protein.

Servings on Maintenance: 2 complex carb servings per day (weight permitting); vegans or vegetarians are allowed up to 3 servings of legumes per day because they serve as a protein.

RADICAL CARBOHYDRATES (STARCHY VEGETABLES, LEGUMES & GRAINS)

Beetroot (85g)
Carrots (cooked) (80g)
Parsnips (80g)
Peas (80g)
*Swede (85g)
Squash (winter) (100g)
Sweet potato 1 small
*Turnip (80g)
Yam 1 small

Tigernuts, tigernut flour, horchata (handful tigernuts or 240ml horchata)
Millet (90g cooked)
White basmati rice (80g cooked)
Sorghum (85g cooked)
Adzuki beans (115g cooked)
Black beans (85g cooked)

Butter beans (95g cooked)
Cannellini beans (90g cooked)
Chickpeas (garbanzo beans) (80g cooked)
Kidney beans (90g cooked)
Lentils (100g cooked)

DAIRY (IF TOLERATED)

Dive into dairy with caution. Many folks are casein and lactose intolerant, so cheese and milk are off limits. Casein is a protein in milk, and casein sensitivities often accompany gluten sensitivities. Many almond-, rice-, and soy-based cheeses also contain casein, so check labels. Even those with dairy sensitivities may be able to eat dairy-based yogurt because the lactose is predigested in the fermentation process—but the casein remains. Butter, cream, and ghee, on the other hand, are digested as fats. The best dairy products are pasture-raised, organic, raw, and fermented for the probiotic benefits (see next section, "Prebiotics & Probiotics"). Look for raw, properly aged artisan cheeses, aged six months or more.

When it comes to fermented (cultured) dairy, you can't assume yogurt, sour cream, cream cheese, and so on contain live cultures: Look for the ones that do. Many commercial varieties are pasteurized and everything is killed off, which is not helpful in any way. Always select those with active, live cultures—or make your own!

RADICAL TIPS: DAIRY

- Full-fat Greek yogurt or cream combined with fruits makes a refreshing dessert. If dairy is a no-go, then substitute unsweetened coconut yogurt or coconut cream—and now there is even cashew yogurt! Either way, top with toasted flax, hemp hearts, chia seeds, or shredded unsweetened coconut for crunch, a boost of fiber, and some omega power.

- A great new product on the market is coconut cheese, which is made using coconut oil. That may sound a bit weird but it actually tastes very cheeselike, and nothing like the flavor of coconut!

Servings: If tolerated, 1 to 2 servings per day.

DAIRY

Butter (1 tablespoon)	Kefir (240ml)	Sour cream (2 tablespoons)
Buttermilk (240ml)	Ghee (1 tablespoon)	Swiss cheese (30g)
Cottage cheese (115g)	Goat cheese (30g)	Yogurt (225g)
Cheddar (30g)	Gouda (30g)	Coconut cheese (1–2 slices)
Cream (1 tablespoon)	Lassi (240ml)	Cashew yogurt or coconut yogurt (if dairy intolerant) (225g)
Cream cheese (2 tablespoons)	Milk (raw) (240ml)	
Edam cheese (30g)	Mozzarella (30g)	
Feta (30g)	Parmesan (30g)	
	Ricotta (115g)	

PREBIOTICS & PROBIOTICS

Probiotic foods are those selectively fermented with bacteria that are beneficial for your gut. If you take probiotics but don't nurture those organisms, you're wasting time—like adopting a pet and then not feeding it. *Your microbiome will not flourish without prebiotics.* Prebiotics are special food-derived fibers that feed these beneficial bacteria. Probiotics and prebiotics work together to optimize the balance and diversity of your microbiome, which is why many probiotic supplements contain prebiotics as well. Good prebiotic and probiotic intake is necessary for a healthy body weight, good digestion, low cardiovascular risk, and minimal inflammation.

You can take a probiotic supplement, but an even better option is eating traditionally fermented foods with live cultures, such as sauerkraut. Fermented foods help your body produce acetylcholine, a neurotransmitter. Within the context of digestion, acetylcholine prevents constipation by stimulating movement of the bowel and increasing the release of digestive enzymes from your stomach, pancreas, and gallbladder. When used regularly, sauerkraut and its juice (brine) improve bile production.

If you tolerate dairy, fermented dairy is another great probiotic superfood. Make sure you either make your own or you select commercial products made from cultured raw, organic grass-fed milk—and not loaded up with sugar. High-quality fermented dairy also provides valuable protein, calcium, B vitamins, and even cancer-fighting conjugated linoleic acid (CLA).

RADICAL TIPS: PROBIOTICS AND PREBIOTICS

- Have your yogurt on some cucumber or jicama (yam bean) sticks or smeared over an underripe banana.
- Some brands offer a variety of cultured dairy beyond just yogurt, including sour cream, kefir, cottage cheese, and cream cheese. The best place to find them is in the refrigerated section of your favorite natural food market.
- Making your own fermented vegetables and cultured dairy is simple, cost-effective, and fun!' Valerie Burke has a nice guide to making fermented pickles and sauerkraut on her blog.[8]
- The brine from sauerkraut is a digestive tonic on its own and can be used as a substitute for digestive bitters. Start slowly with 1 teaspoon and work your way up to a few tablespoons, several times a day.
- Umeboshi plum vinegar is a

delightfully tasty vinegar with prebiotic benefits.

- Try sneaking a little probiotic into each meal. For example, add a teaspoon of miso to your bowl of soup just prior to serving, or toss a couple of tablespoons of sauerkraut to your salad or cooked veggies. Instead of vinegar or lemon juice, try making your salad dressing using sauerkraut brine. A dollop of yogurt or cultured sour cream makes a tasty topper for cooked veggies. Toss a few spoonfuls of fermented veggies into your guacamole!

Probiotic servings: 1 to 5 servings per day, starting slowly and increasing as tolerated (a probiotic supplement counts as 1 serving).

Prebiotic food servings: Incorporate prebiotic foods into daily meals as often as possible.

PROBIOTIC FOODS

Cultured dairy (sour cream, yogurt, cottage cheese, kefir, lassi, etc. with live cultures)
Cashew yogurt
Miso
Fermented vegetables (sauerkraut, naturally fermented pickles, kimchi, kvass)
Fermented vegetable brine (1 teaspoon to 2 tablespoons)

PREBIOTIC FOODS

Many prebiotic foods double as bitters . . . notice all the asterisks in the list below!

*Asparagus, raw
Bananas, underripe
*Chicory root, raw
*Cocoa or cacao
*Dandelion greens
Flaxseed
*Garlic
Glucomannan fiber (konjac root, used in shirataki noodles [branded as Miracle Noodles])
*Jerusalem artichoke, raw
*Jicama (yam beans)
*Leeks, raw
Miso
*Seaweed
Tigernuts and horchata (a beverage made from tigernuts)
Umeboshi plum and its vinegar
Yacón

SUGAR & SPICE & EVERYTHING NICE IN YOUR PANTRY

Herbs and spices transform even the simplest meal by adding real soul to your food. However, the Radical Metabolism–recommended seasonings are not just flavor fixers—they are heavy-duty metabolism enhancers. The antioxidants abundant in these seasonings are synonymous with good health and a trim waistline. They neutralize harmful free radicals in the body, aid the digestive process, support your liver, and protect you from disease.

Spices can offer surprising health benefits. For example, certain spices may help prevent or repair damage from peroxynitrites. Peroxynitrites are unstable ions produced by exposure to mobile phone and Wi-Fi radiation, and they create free radicals that impair your mitochondrial function. Spices, such as cloves, rosemary, turmeric, cinnamon, and ginger, have been scientifically shown to afford protection against peroxynitrite-induced damage.[9]

Let's take a look at a few of the most powerful Radical Metabolism herbs and spices.

*HORSERADISH

Hats off to horseradish—it's a bitter! That means it's good for your bile and gallbladder. Not only does the aroma of this superfood knock your socks off, but it has ten times the cancer-fighting power of broccoli, thanks to chemoprotective compounds called glucosinolates that flip on cancer-fighting genes in your body.[10] Horseradish also has benefits for your respiratory system (chest congestion, sinus infections, tonsillitis, colds, and flu), urinary tract infections, joint and muscle pain, and headaches, and assists with detoxification. It's very easy to grow in your garden—but don't plant more than one or it will totally take over! Prepared horseradish is an option, keeping in mind that organic is always preferable.

CAYENNE

Cayenne pepper's heat comes from capsicum, which increases the body's metabolic rate and cleans fat out of the arteries. An Oxford study found cayenne pepper produced a 20 percent jump in metabolism! Cayenne does so much more than create a tongue-tingling meal—it's loaded with B vitamins and vitamins A, D, and E, as well as calcium, phosphorous, and iron. It is high in immune-boosting beta-carotene and is used as a painkiller, antiseptic, and digestive aid. It adds a real kick to all your veggies, sauces, dips, and soups. I even like a pinch of this hot stuff in my smoothie. Cayenne is a nightshade, so if you're sensitive to nightshades, you might want to skip this one. I just wanted to include it for its admirable nutritional qualities.

*CINNAMON

Cinnamon is your blood sugar's best friend and can reduce the glycemic impact of a meal by almost 30 percent. I recommend only Ceylon cinnamon because most commercial cinnamons contain the liver-damaging ingredient coumarin that can be harmful to health when taken in excess. Try Ceylon cinnamon in desserts, lamb, coffee, tea, and smoothies.

CUMIN

This peppery biblical spice is a wonderful taste enhancer and catalyst for weight loss. The latest research out of the Middle East, where cumin is popularly consumed, shows that 1 teaspoon can boost weight loss by 50 percent, mostly due to its thermogenic effects. This is a superspice for hummus, beans, chili, and any Mexican dish.

*GINGER

Ginger increases the thermic effect of food, giving your metabolic engines a boost so you'll burn more calories. According to an Australian study, ginger can increase metabolism as much as 20 percent. A compound in ginger called gingerol has natural appetite suppressant properties by raising your leptin level. Ginger also suppresses cortisol production, and cortisol is known to promote fat storage. Ginger revs circulation and promotes healthy sweating, encouraging detoxification. It supports liver function, clears up clogged arteries, and lowers serum cholesterol levels. It is effective for motion sickness and nausea. Ginger is tasty on salmon and lends itself well to cookies (I just love ginger snaps), puddings, and custards. Try a cup of ginger tea— just ½ to ¾ teaspoon of ground ginger in hot water, with or without a squeeze of lemon.

MUSTARD

Mustard is a must in my kitchen. In the dried, powdered state or as a prepared mustard spread, it provides a burst of tangy spiciness while kicking your metabolism into high gear. Study data from Oxford Polytechnic Institute shows that mustard spikes metabolic rates by 25 percent—by adding mustard to a meal, participants burned at least 45 extra calories over the next three hours. Try a pinch of dried mustard in your homemade salad dressings, mayo, pickles, and even soup.

REAL SEA SALT

Don't be afraid to salt your food! Numerous studies have refuted the myth that high-salt diets increase your risk of heart disease and cause high blood pressure. Not only that, but sea salt may kick your metabolism up a notch! A recent animal study showed a high-salt diet actually *increased metabolism*, causing the animals to eat 25 percent more calories just to maintain their weight.[11] Just make sure it's genuine sea salt you're using, not the laboratory-concocted chemical sodium chloride variety.

> *Myth: Salt drives up blood pressure and increases heart attack risk.*

*TURMERIC

You almost can't go anywhere these days without seeing something about turmeric, the superstar of many popular curries. This exotic yellow spice owes its high antioxidant content to curcumin, its most active compound. What you may not have heard about this special spice is that it can help thin and decongest the bile so your body can metabolize fat more efficiently. Turmeric can be added to curries, beans, meat stews, fish dinners, and soups. It's the best spice for a barbecue because adding turmeric to meats before they are grilled reduces toxic compounds up to 40 percent.

RADICAL TIPS: SPICES

- Sprinkle Radical Metabolism seasonings onto your meals to jump-start fat burning! A few suggestions are basil, caraway, cayenne, coriander, mustard, turmeric, ginger, Ceylon cinnamon, dill, garlic, parsley, and cumin.
- Add a dab of horseradish to cultured sour cream for a delightful beef or bison dipping sauce.

HERBS, SPICES, SEASONINGS & PANTRY STAPLES

Anise	*Cinnamon (Ceylonese)	*Ginger
*Basil	Cloves	*Horseradish
Bay leaves	*Coriander	*Mint
Black pepper	Cumin	Mustard, dry
*Caraway seeds	Curry	Nutmeg
Cardamom	*Dill	Oregano
Cayenne (nightshade)	Fennel	Paprika, regular and
Chipotle powder	*Fenugreek seeds	smoked (nightshade)
(nightshade)	*Garlic	*Parsley

Rosemary
*Saffron
Sea salt
*Sesame seeds
Tarragon
Thyme
*Turmeric
Agar-agar
Arrowroot
Aluminum-free baking
   powder
Apple cider vinegar

Umeboshi plum
   vinegar
Balsamic vinegar (only
   from Modena, Italy)
*Bitter chocolate and
   cacao (look for 65%
   to 85% cacao)
Capers
Dijon mustard
Extracts (vanilla,
   almond, lemon,
   peppermint)

Miso
*Seaweed flakes (dulse,
   arame, nori, kombu,
   wakame, etc.)
Sriracha sauce
   (nightshade)
Tamari (gluten-free)
Coconut aminos
Fish sauce

SWEETENERS

Research is mounting that sugar is a major culprit in diseases such as obesity, diabetes, and dementia, according to Dr. Robert Lustig, author of *Fat Chance: Beating the Odds Against Sugar, Processed Food, Obesity, and Disease.* The latest in a long string of studies about the link between sugar and metabolic syndrome shows *causation*—not just association.[12] If sugar is a nutritional bomb, then glucose-fructose syrup/high-fructose corn syrup is the nuclear version! Concentrated fructose raises blood pressure, damages the kidneys, drives up inflammation, and is quite literally cancer's favorite food.

As bad as refined sugars are, artificial sweeteners, such as aspartame and sucralose, *are even worse!* We need sweeteners that do not raise our levels of fat-packing insulin—and there aren't many that don't have detrimental health effects of one kind or another. The following are my top four go-to sweeteners. Just keep in mind that part of this plan is to *retrain your palate* to love bitter flavors as much as sweet, so the more you can decrease sweeteners over time, the better.

STEVIA, THE WONDER HERB

Stevia is a versatile herb that can be used in place of sugar for baking, smoothies, and beverages without raising your blood sugar. This low-glycemic sweetener imparts sweetness with zero calories and zero carbs. Stevia is thirty times sweeter than sugar so a little goes a long way. When a recipe calls for one teaspoon of sugar, use ⅓ teaspoon of stevia instead.

YACÓN SYRUP

Yacón syrup comes from yacón root, a tuber that's naturally high in prebiotics, including inulin and fructooligosaccharides (FOS). Unlike most roots, which are quite starchy, yacón stores its sugars as FOS rather than starch, which accounts for its sweeter taste. In fact, yacón is thought to be the richest source of FOS in the natural world. And happily, it scores a measly 1 on the glycemic index, which is the same as erythritol and inulin. (Stevia and monk fruit are zeros.)[13]

Fructooligosaccharides resist breakdown by your digestive enzymes so they reach your colon intact and act as a prebiotic for your gut flora. Yacón also bulks up the stool, improves gastric emptying, decreases food cravings, and reduces fat accumulation in the liver. Studies show yacón can improve body mass index (BMI), insulin, and LDL levels.[14] Yacón syrup (sometimes called yacón nectar) can be found in many nutrition stores or ordered online. Make sure you purchase pure, raw, organic yacón that is free of additives. When the syrup is thermally processed, much of its FOS converts to sugar, so you lose a large part of its nutritional value. To qualify as "raw," the processing temperatures must not exceed about 40°C (104°F).

Yacón syrup is delightful in beverages and salad dressings. Its flavor profile mingles particularly nicely with apple cider vinegar.

CHICORY ROOT

Chicory root is used to make a natural clean-tasting sweetener whose carbohydrates are indigestible, so they pass right through your digestive tract with a zero-calorie impact. Even better is that chicory root is a prebiotic—it feeds your friendly gut bugs!

MONK FRUIT

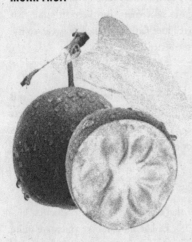

Another healthy sweetener option is monk fruit (*luo han guo*, or *lo han*, which comes from China and is actually part of the gourd family). Since your body metabolizes monk fruit differently, it will not raise your insulin and is safe for diabetics, perfect for adding to teas and smoothies. The only downside is its cost, due to export restrictions and the expense of its complicated extraction process.

Monk fruit is intensely sweet, ten times sweeter than stevia—three hundred times sweeter than sugar—but its sweetness isn't due to natural sugars.

Instead, it contains powerful antioxidants called mogrosides, which taste sweet but are metabolized differently than sugar. Monk fruit has a long history of benefits for diabetics from its positive effects on pancreatic cells to improve insulin sensitivity. Monk fruit is known as the longevity fruit for its wide-ranging health benefits in fighting free radicals, lowering inflammation, combating infections, relieving fatigue, and possibly preventing cancer. It's also a natural antihistamine. Make sure your monk fruit sweetener is not combined with other agents, such as sugar alcohols. Always read those labels.

WHAT ABOUT THE SUGAR ALCOHOLS?

Sugar alcohols, such as xylitol, sorbitol, and erythritol, are carbohydrates with characteristics of both a sugar and an alcohol. They have become popular due to their low glycemic index, but are they safe? The latest science is discouraging.

Evidence is mounting that *all* sugar alcohols are disruptive to your microbiome, from your mouth all the way down to your gut. Therefore, I can no longer recommend them—even erythritol. Erythritol is commercially manufactured by fermenting cornstarch with yeast, typically genetically engineered yeast.[15]

> *Myth: Sugar alcohols, such as xylitol and erythritol, are completely safe.*

SWEETENERS

Stevia	Monk fruit (luo han guo/lo han)
Raw yacón syrup (a.k.a. yacón nectar)	Pure maple syrup (in small amounts)
Chicory root	Coconut sugar/coconut blossom nectar

BEVERAGES

WATER

It all starts with water. As the purest detox and diluting agent, water can take the edge off your appetite, ensure normal bowel and kidney function, rid your body of wastes, and alleviate fluid retention. Consuming 1.5 to 2 litres of water each day will help your liver metabolize stored fat into energy. Drinking cold water will enhance metabolism, while dehydration kicks up cortisol, resulting in more tummy fat. It's best to drink before or between meals to avoid diluting gastric juices.

Servings: Drink 1.5 to 2 litres per day (water and herbal teas), in between meals to avoid diluting gastric juices.

*COFFEE

Gone are the days when coffee had to shoulder the blame for heart disease, ulcers, and nervous disorders. Not only does coffee not cause those problems, but recent studies show that coffee beans improve insulin sensitivity and metabolic rate, and their antioxidant compounds reduce LDLs and inflammatory markers. Coffee lowers your risk for heart disease and colorectal cancer, protects against neurodegenerative conditions, including Parkinson's and Alzheimer's, and reduces pain—along with many other health benefits. Even coffee implants (rectal, vaginal, penal, and oral) are being used to treat fibroid tumors, ovarian cysts, infections, adhesions, and more. *Even better, it's a bitter*—happy dance! To quote Dr. Mark Circus, "It will take nothing short of another mass extinction event to curb our love of coffee."[16] The only caveats are to make sure your cuppa Joe is organically produced and not grown in a torrent of pesticides, and be careful about coffee if you have adrenal issues.

Coffee has several polyphenols and other compounds that are exceedingly beneficial to metabolism. A 2017 rat study demonstrated coffee's positive benefits for metabolic syndrome. Rats fed a mixture of coffee compounds (caffeic acid, trigonelline, and cafestol) experienced improved insulin sensitivity and reduced levels of fat in their liver.[17] Coffee beans have another secret weapon—chlorogenic acid, which is the most abundant polyphenol in coffee. Chlorogenic acid, or CGA, is thermogenic, so it instructs your body's fat cells to burn their fatty acids for fuel. Research published in the *American Journal of Clinical Nutrition* found CGA to reduce blood sugar fluctuations by 50 percent after just five days.[18]

CGA can stimulate weight loss, boost energy, and slash your risk for diabetes and heart disease. This powerful polyphenol even helps individuals fall asleep faster, which is surprising for something in coffee (which is not to suggest that the caffeine won't erase this effect). CGA also ramps up fat burning while you're bagging your zzz's. A Norwegian study reported that women who drank high-CGA coffee dropped three times more weight than women who consumed lower CGA brews. The average cuppa Joe contains about 130 milligrams of CGA, but you need *eight times that* to reap its benefits. How can you boost CGA?

Chlorogenic acid levels depend on where coffee beans originate and how they're roasted. Coffee plants grown at high altitudes with extreme climatic conditions (temperature fluctuations, wind, etc.) will produce more polyphenols to protect themselves. Look for beans from Ethiopia, Kenya, Mexico, Colombia, and Brazil, especially higher elevations.

If you're a dark roast fan, you may want to dial it down a notch to medium or even light. Once beans are roasted beyond medium, they've lost 75 percent of their fat-blasting, waistline-reducing polyphenols. Learn to enjoy your brew sans dairy because it makes polyphenols 28 percent less bioavailable. What about decaf? Even the best ones have 25 percent fewer polyphenols.

Servings: One cup of coffee per day.

OOLONG TEA

Oolong's weight-loss benefits are well established by science. If you have thyroid concerns, I would avoid oolong due to potential fluoride contamination.

Servings: Two cups per day.

ROASTED DANDELION ROOT TEA

A herbal tea with earthy notes, roasted dandelion root is a slimming and caffeine-free alternative to coffee. Especially effective as a liver tonic, dandy tea can help lower elevated liver enzymes for those who have overdone alcohol, sugar, trans fats, and medications. Try adding a tablespoon of coconut oil as a great way to begin your day with metabolism-boosting healthy fats.

HIBISCUS TEA

Hot or iced, hibiscus tea will hydrate you and flush toxins and excess fluids out of your body, due to its diuretic properties. Hibiscus has also been shown to reduce high blood pressure, thanks to its anti-inflammatory properties, and to reduce high cholesterol, thanks to its antioxidant content. Sip it to stay healthy during cold and flu season, as its rich ascorbic acid content helps strengthen your immune system. Hibiscus tea is also thought to help relieve menstrual pain and lift your mood.

ROOIBOS TEA

Rooibos is a South African herb rich in health-promoting polyphenolic antioxidants, and because the tea is made from tender young leaves, it's low in fluoride. Rooibos is the only known source of a beneficial and rare antioxidant called aspalathin. Rooibos is also known to significantly boost superoxide dismutase (SOD), one of the body's most powerful antioxidant enzymes inside and outside cell membranes.[19] SOD combats free radicals and reduces inflammation. Unfermented (green) rooibos has higher levels of antioxidants than does traditional fermented rooibos. This herbal tea is also free of caffeine, oxalates, and tannins, so it's the perfect Radical Metabolism tea!

ORGANIC BONE BROTHS

Bone broths make a lovely warming beverage, especially in the winter . . . more than a beverage but less than a meal. Additions such as your favorite omega-rich oils (hemp, sesame, pine nut, etc.) and thermogenic spices can be added for health-boosting effects and character. Try a mug with a splash of lemon! In Maintenance, a splash of coconut milk is divine.

ALCOHOLIC BEVERAGES

These are best avoided. Not only does alcohol place an extra burden on your liver, but my clinical experience has convinced me that even moderate alcohol consumption has a profound influence on women's inability to lose weight. This is largely due to its effect of elevating estrogen levels, which is well documented by science. This is significant because so many women trying to lose weight are already estrogen dominant—and this just adds to the problem. Alcohol may also be linked to decreased progesterone levels in premenopausal women.[20] The one exception to the alcohol rule is the use of dark non-GMO beer as a meat marinade, and of course the alcohol is completely cooked away during grilling.

BEVERAGES

*Coffee	Meadowsweet herb tea
Oolong tea	Pau d-arco tea
Limit coffee to one cup per day	*Peppermint tea
and oolong tea to two cups	Rosemary tea
Water	Organic non-GMO dark beer
Hibiscus tea	*Angostura bitters
*Roasted dandelion root tea	Bone broths
Chicory root tea	Unsweetened cranberry juice
*Ginger tea	

TOP 20 TIPS FOR RADICAL SUCCESS

1. **Start with a RADICAL pantry raid.** When you sort through that toxic cookware, toss out the toxic foods as well. Restock your fridge, freezer, and pantry with wholesome radical foods. Say good-bye to overprocessed, overheated, prepackaged foods.
2. **Start slowly.** When starting a new food or supplement, always start slowly to see how you react. Start only one new food at a time so if you do have a reaction, you'll know what did it.
3. **Plan ahead.** There is great truth to the adage that "failing to plan is planning to fail." Plan your meals one to two weeks in advance. If you work, spend a day or two preparing meals for the week. For example, assemble some slow cooker meals so all you have to do in the morning is dump it in and turn it on. Be sure to prep some healthy "convenience

HEALTHY EQUIVALENTS & SWAPS

FOODS TO LOSE	FOODS TO USE
1 tablespoon sugar	1 tablespoon pure maple syrup or coconut sugar
1 square or 30g unsweetened dark chocolate	3 tablespoons raw cacao or carob powder plus 1 tablespoon water plus 1 tablespoon sesame oil
Breadcrumbs	Ground flax seeds, ground chia seeds, ground nuts
Sauce and soup thickeners	Arrowroot, ground chia seeds
1 tablespoon margarine or cooking oil	*1 tablespoon pastured butter or 3 tablespoons ground flaxseeds

*Baked goods with flaxseed will brown more quickly, therefore either shorten the baking time or lower oven temperature by 10°C/25°F.

MISCELLANEOUS EQUIVALENTS

IF YOU DON'T HAVE THIS:	USE THIS:
Garlic, 1 clove, fresh	⅛ teaspoon garlic powder
Ginger, 1 teaspoon, grated fresh	¼ teaspoon ground ginger
Herb, 1 tablespoon fresh	½ to 1 teaspoon crushed dried herb
Herb, 1 teaspoon fresh	½ teaspoon ground dried herb
Onion, 1 small	1 teaspoon onion powder or 1 tablespoon dried minced onion

HEALTHY FAT EQUIVALENTS

EACH OF THE FOLLOWING IS THE EQUIVALENT OF ONE TABLESPOON OF THE HEALTHY FATS OR OILS.

1 tablespoon homemade mayo
2 tablespoons nut or seed butter (almond, cashew, pumpkin, sesame)
Nuts: 7 almonds, 2 medium Brazil nuts, 4 walnut halves, 6 cashews, 4 pecan halves, 3 macadamia nuts, 15 pistachios, 2 tablespoons pine nuts
1 tablespoon butter or ghee (clarified butter)
1 tablespoon seeds (pumpkin, chia, sesame, sunflower, hemp)
3 tablespoons ground toasted flaxseeds
2 teaspoons sour cream or 1 tablespoon heavy cream
Coconut: 2 tablespoons shredded coconut OR 6 tablespoons (90ml) coconut milk OR 1 tablespoon coconut cream or coconut manna (coconut butter)
¼ small avocado
8 large olives
30g sacha inchi seeds
3 anchovy fillets
All products should be organic, full fat, and come from grass-pastured animals.

foods" as well, for grab-and-go. Make more than you need and make friends with leftovers—twice the food for the same amount of work.

4. **Get the whole family on board.** Even if they aren't strictly doing the program (although I hope they are), this is a great opportunity to help them clean up their diet up a bit.

5. **Be the mad scientist.** Remember—*you are the alchemist.* Have fun experimenting in the kitchen!

6. **Go to farmer's markets.** Get in the habit of frequenting farmer's markets in your area. Stock up on organic fruits and vegetables, focusing on what's in season in your area. Local farms and food markets are producing wonderful products from artisan cheeses to sauerkraut and kimchi, homemade jerky, probiotic beverages, and everything in between.

7. **Get sixy.** Don't be afraid of those omega-6s! Omega-6 parent oils (unadulterated sources of linoleic acid) in the form of sprouted seeds, nuts, hemp oil, and others are necessary to restore cell membranes and reignite your metabolic fires.

8. **Hemp is heavenly.** Experiment with omega-rich balanced hemp oil on salads, a tablespoon or two of nutty hemp hearts. Hemp contains an almost ideal omega-6 to omega-3 ratio. Just treat hemp hearts with TLC—always store them in the fridge and use them up quickly.

9. **Change up your cooking oils.** Ghee is a great fat for cooking because it has a higher smoke point than butter, and some heat-tolerant omega-6s, to boot. Bone broth is also excellent for higher-heat cooking. On the 21-Day Reboot, stick to those two. Then, when you start the Maintenance phase, you can add neutral oils, such as macadamia nut, avocado, coconut, etc., with appropriate smoke points for the task. By *neutral*, I mean they don't throw off your omega ratio or compete for space in cell membranes.

10. **Butter is back.** Butter up those veggies with organic pastured butter. Butter from pasture-raised cows is rich in both omega-6s and omega-3s.

11. **Go nuts.** Nuts are a rich source of omega-6s, and to a lesser degree omega-3s. Pecans, walnuts, and cashews can be used in place of bread crumbs and binders in recipes. Snack on nut butters (pumpkin, almond, sesame, cashew, walnut) with celery, carrot, and cucumber sticks, or slather onto a Granny Smith apple between meals. Pine nuts are delicious tossed into all types of tomato sauce, and toasted crushed pistachios make a nice breading for chicken and fish. Note once again that I cannot in good conscience recommend any almond products produced in the USA,

whether organic or not, because all almonds are either gassed or overly heated, which negates their nutritional benefits. The "King of Nuts" has sadly fallen off the throne. Seek out Spanish almonds, if possible.

12. **Breakfast suggestions:** How about a smoothie with kefir or yogurt, or chia seed pudding with hempseed milk and berries?

13. **Bitters and Metabolixirs:** Don't forget those daily bitters! Boost your digestion and ramp up your metabolism with bitters and Metabolixirs. The Metabolixirs can be added *after* the 21-Day Radical Reboot.

14. **An eggs-cellent egg substitute:** It is best to avoid eggs due to gallbladder sensitivities, so you'll need an egg substitute for your recipes. Here's a simple one that really works! To replace one egg, blend 1 tablespoon of ground flaxseed with 3 tablespoons water and let stand for three minutes before adding to a recipe.

15. **Fun with coconut.** Once you finish the Reboot and move on to the Maintenance phase, you and your old friend coconut can have your reunion! Coconut oil is a "neutral" metabolism-friendly fat that won't compete with the omegas, so you can safely add it back to your diet. Add a little to your coffee or juice in the morning to get a bit more spring in your step. About 100–120ml of coconut milk or coconut cream in soups or curries creates a wonderfully smooth texture and flavor. Coconut "manna" (coconut butter) is now widely available, which is a combination of coconut oil and coconut cream—and it's scrumptious right off the spoon, or paired with nut butter.

16. **Radical sleep tips:** Sleeping in a cooler room has significant fat-burning benefits because it increases your body's brown fat, which ramps up metabolism. Setting your thermostat between 15 and 20°C (60–68°F) is optimal.[21] Getting the right amount of sleep is important, too. Those who sleep 8.5 hours per night are found to burn 400 more calories every day than those who get only 5.5 hours of nightly zzz's.

17. **Give fasting a try.** Intermittent fasting has been shown to produce metabolic benefits by boosting your body's production of human growth hormone and retraining your body to burn fat for fuel. If you're concerned about being hungry, studies suggest this is not typically experienced. Hunger passes quickly because the hunger hormone ghrelin peaks within two days and declines thereafter. There are many types of intermittent fasting, so feel free to experiment! For example, confine your eating between 10 a.m. and 6 p.m., or between noon and 8 p.m.—whatever works best for your schedule and lifestyle.

18. **Detox isn't fun but it passes.** Realize that you *might* feel worse before you feel better—your body may be doing some long-overdue detox. *This is a good sign and it will pass!*

19. **Remember your why.** If you fall off the wagon, dust yourself off and hop back on! Don't quit—just make adjustments.

20. **This is not a diet!** Think of it as a road map to becoming the ridiculously lean, healthy, and ageless person you deserve to be!

RADICAL REBOOT FAQS

Here are some common questions people have as they prepare to launch into the 21-Day Radical Reboot.

Q: Do I have to discontinue my current supplements when I start the 21-Day Radical Reboot?

A: Your core supplements will likely be fairly similar to those on the Radical Metabolism program. Keep taking your multivitamins, minerals, vitamin D, probiotics, and so on. If you're on CLA or GLA, please continue because those are über-omega-6s.

Q: What if I can't eat dairy?

A: If you don't tolerate dairy, make sure you include some fermented vegetables, such as sauerkraut, kimchi, naturally cultured pickles, and so on, for those valuable probiotics. Consider adding a probiotic supplement as well. A newer dairy alternative is cashew yogurt, as well as coconut yogurt, which you can have once you're on maintenance. If you *do* tolerate dairy, replace ordinary dairy products with raw cultured dairy from animals raised on pasture—such as yogurt, kefir, raw cheese, cultured butter, and sour cream—this way, you get your naturally occurring omegas and probiotics all in one. Whatever you choose, top it off with some crunchy seeds, crushed nuts, or shredded coconut (maintenance only) for a nice little crunch.

Q: What if I've been on Fat Flush?

A: The two programs are completely compatible. You can use the 4-Day Radical Intensive as a cleanse between Fat Flush Phases 1 and 2, and 2 and 3. You can implement the 21-Day Radical Reboot in Phase 2 or 3. Simply use the 21-Day Radical Reboot to add variety to your Phase 3 regimen with new oils, radical carbs, and yummy prebiotics. I would do Phase 3 Fat Flush for a week, then switch to Radical Metabolism for a week, and repeat the cycle. No more boredom or reliance on the same foods.

Q: Are there any special accommodations for men?

A: The only adjustment I might make for a man is bumping up the protein servings and adding one more starch (a starchy vegetable, grain, or legume), depending on body weight, activity level, and metabolic variables. If a man has a significant amount of weight to lose, he might want to keep the starches low and just bump up the protein.

10 MENU PLANS

> I am really happy to have been introduced to this. I have been fol-
> lowing your recipes pretty closely, but experimenting with vegetables
> off the bitters list. I bought a juicer right from the start and have
> been making two glasses a day. Love it! Juicing is a little bit of work
> but not too much to dissuade me. I find it's a great way to curb my
> desire for anything sweet.
>
> —Marianne F., age 50

> When completing the 21-day protocol, I was very clear-headed and
> very focused. I loved the food recipes and so did my husband!
>
> —Suzanne K., age 61

You are now ready to launch your new you! Eating the Radical Metabolism way prom-
ises to rev up your metabolism even as you indulge in your favorite foods. The plan
presented below is a simple but tasty 28-day sample menu to get you started. With this
new radical approach, you will see slimming as you replenish your body's omega fat
reserves, thin your bile, improve your gallbladder function, repair your gut, and rejuvenate your mitochondria. Everything you eat and drink will build vitality and strength
and power up fat burning!

You have just finished your 4-day Cleanse and we want to make it easy
on your digestive tract, so you will notice that for the next three weeks your
breakfasts consist of light, easily digestible, but nutrient-dense liquid foods.
You will start each day with the Citrus Blaster we talked about in Chapter 9.
(The recipe is also given on page 201.) These give you a mega-infusion of pure
fat-blasting nutritional goodness. And to coffee lovers everywhere—you're
welcome!

Keep in mind that these menus are not set in stone. Breakfast, lunch, and dinner
are totally interchangeable. Alter them to fit your lifestyle and personal preferences.
The only exception is the Citrus Blaster, which could keep you awake if you drink it

too late in the day. Just stick to the basic radical principles in terms of servings, portion sizes, and food groups so you maintain control over your insulin levels. You can always refer back to Chapter 9 for all the delicious details.

A FEW GUIDING PRINCIPLES

- **Beverages:** Drink at least 1.5 to 2 litres of water and herbal tea, such as hibiscus and roasted dandelion, between meals every day. If you drink oolong tea, remember to limit it to two cups per day and limit coffee to one cup daily (which includes Citrus Blaster).
- **Dairy:** If you don't tolerate dairy, feel free to eliminate it. That said, probiotic foods are extremely important, so if you are unable to tolerate fermented dairy, grab some of those fabulous fermented vegetables, such as dill pickles or sauerkraut, or add a teaspoon of miso to your soup.
- **Vegan options:** If you are vegan or vegetarian, simply substitute tempeh or 80–90g of cooked beans or other legumes for one of the animal proteins each day.
- **Omega fats:** Don't forget to include those all-important omega-6s and -3s with every single meal, which can be as simple as adding a drizzle of hemp oil or sprinkling some ground flaxseeds over your dish.
- **Strange and wonderfully radical new foods:** I have included a select few radical new foods for their stellar health benefits, including umeboshi plum vinegar and Siberian pine nut oil. Umeboshi plum vinegar is tasty and has probiotic benefits, but if you prefer, you can always substitute apple cider vinegar. Pine nut oil is a delicious omega-6 shown to effectively resolve common digestive issues, so I strongly encourage investing in a bottle to try out over the next twenty-eight days.

Now, on to the menu! The menu that follows provides suggestions for four weeks of meals. The first three weeks are the 21-Day Reboot, and the fourth week represents one week on the Maintenance Plan.

On Maintenance, you will add back those other healthy neutral fats and oils, such as avocado, coconut, and olive, as well as eggs and onions as tolerated. On Maintenance, you will also score one to two extra servings of radical carbohydrates and fruits each day. Read on to discover the strategy for reshaping your body and transforming your life in just twenty-eight days.

WEEK 1: 21-DAY RADICAL REBOOT

SUNDAY

Breakfast:
Citrus Blaster (page 201)

Snack:
7 walnuts
1 small apple

Lunch:
115g grilled chicken breast sprinkled with 1 teaspoon ground flaxseeds
Tricolored salad (rocket, radicchio, and endive), with 1 tablespoon hemp oil and
  lemon juice

Mid- to Late Afternoon:
Metabolixir (pages 196–197)

Dinner:
1 (115g) Radical Turkey Burger (page 207)
100g steamed spring greens topped with 1 tablespoon butter or ghee
Small sweet potato, mashed, with cinnamon

Treat:
2 squares bitter dark chocolate

MONDAY

Breakfast:
Citrus Blaster (page 201)

Snack:
Celery and carrot sticks with 1 tablespoon chopped fresh dill and 1 tablespoon
  lemon juice

Lunch:

100g cottage cheese on a bed of butterhead lettuce, sliced cucumber and red peppers with 1 tablespoon Sixy Sesame Salad Dressing (page 221) and 1 tablespoon of chia seeds

80g pineapple

Mid- to Late Afternoon:

Metabolixir (pages 196–197)

Dinner:

115g grilled wild-caught salmon drizzled with hemp oil and lemon juice

80g peas with mint

Creamy Dreamy Watercress Soup (pages 218–219)

Treat:

15 pistachios

TUESDAY

Breakfast:

Citrus Blaster (page 201)

Snack:

7 walnuts

Lunch:

1 (115g) grilled beef patty with mustard and cumin

Grapefruit Slaw (page 214) sprinkled with 1 tablespoon ground toasted flaxseeds

---

Mid- to Late Afternoon:

Metabolixir (pages 196–197)

Dinner:

Chicken Schnitzel with Cucumber Salad (pages 206–207)

80g steamed broccoli drizzled with umeboshi plum vinegar and 1 tablespoon pine nut oil

Treat:
240ml Val's Horchata (page 200)

WEDNESDAY

Breakfast:
Citrus Blaster (page 201)

Snack:
1 small pear with 2 tablespoons almond butter

Lunch:
115g canned tuna or salmon with lemon juice and 1 tablespoon hemp oil on bed
of mixed greens and chopped celery sprinkled with 1 tablespoon ground toasted
flaxseeds

Mid- to Late Afternoon:
Metabolixir (pages 196–197)

Dinner:
1 (115g) grilled steak with garlic and rosemary
Steamed artichoke with 1 tablespoon Horseradish Vinaigrette (page 224)
80g roasted root vegetable with 1 tablespoon butter or ghee

Treat:
Two squares bitter dark chocolate

THURSDAY

Breakfast:
Citrus Blaster (page 201)

Snack:
Celery sticks with 2 tablespoons cashew butter and 1 tablespoon ground toasted
flaxseeds

Lunch:

1 (115g) bison or beef burger with dill pickle and mustard on bed of red leaf lettuce, shredded carrot, and radish, with 1 tablespoon Umeboshi Plum Vinaigrette (page 223)

Mid- to Late Afternoon:

Metabolixir (pages 196–197)

Dinner:

1 Melissa's Turkey Sausage Patty (page 203)
80g cooked basmati rice drizzled with 1 tablespoon hempseed oil
Green beans sautéed in Bone Broth (page 216) sprinkled with 1 tablespoon chopped walnuts

Treat:

3 macadamia nuts
1 tangerine

FRIDAY

Breakfast:

Citrus Blaster (page 201)

Snack:

6 cashews

Lunch:

115g tempeh plus garlic, water chestnuts, bok choy, bamboo shoots, and sugarsnap peas stir-fried together in 2 tablespoons Bone Broth (page 216), 1 tablespoon coconut aminos, and ¼ teaspoon ground ginger, topped with 1 tablespoon flaxseed oil

Mid- to Late Afternoon:

Metabolixir (pages 196–197)

Dinner:
Moroccan Chicken (page 209)
100g oven-roasted butternut squash with ginger drizzled with 1 tablespoon pine
  nut oil
2 medium apricots

Treat:
15 pistachios

SATURDAY

Breakfast:
Citrus Blaster (page 201)

Snack:
100g peeled and chopped jicama (yam bean), Jerusalem artichoke or cucumber
  sticks dipped in lime juice, cumin, and 1 tablespoon chia seeds
80g mango

Lunch:
Grilled chicken breast with tarragon and parsley on steamed green beans, topped
  with 1 tablespoon flaxseed oil

Mid- to Late Afternoon:
Metabolixir (pages 196–197)

Dinner:
115g grilled lamb chops marinated in garlic, dried mustard, rosemary, and lemon
  juice
Spaghetti squash drizzled with 1 tablespoon butter or ghee

Treat:
1 Hemp Cacao Magic 6-Ball (page 227)

WEEK 2: 21-DAY RADICAL REBOOT

SUNDAY

Breakfast:
Citrus Blaster (page 201)

Snack:
2 tablespoons sunflower seeds
⅛ cantaloupe melon

Lunch:
115g sardines, chopped celery, chopped parsley, tossed in 1 tablespoon Horseradish
  Vinaigrette (page 224) and topped with 1 tablespoon ground toasted flaxseeds
Creamy Dreamy Watercress Soup (pages 218–219)

Mid- to Late Afternoon:
Metabolixir (pages 196–197)

Dinner:
115g Lemon Garlic Roasted Chicken (page 211)
Roasted asparagus with lemon zest and sesame seeds
90g cooked millet drizzled with 1 tablespoon pine nut oil

Treat:
1 Radical Chocolate Chip Cookie (pages 227–228)

MONDAY

Breakfast:
Citrus Blaster (page 201)

Snack:
1 (single-serving) package roasted seaweed snacks
2 medium plums

Lunch:
Chicken bowl made with 115g chopped grilled chicken mixed with sliced radishes, watercress, celery, parsley, and 1 tablespoon Horseradish Vinaigrette (page 224) sprinkled with 1 tablespoon hemp hearts

Mid- to Late Afternoon:
Metabolixir (pages 196–197)

Dinner:
240ml Creamy Dreamy Watercress Soup (pages 218–219)
Teriyaki Tempeh (page 212)
80g roasted carrots with 1 tablespoon butter or ghee and dill

Treat:
4 walnuts with 2 squares bitter dark chocolate

TUESDAY

Breakfast:
Citrus Blaster (page 201)

Snack:
100g peeled and roughly chopped jicama (yam beans), Jerusalem artichokes or cucumber in 250g Greek yogurt, topped with 1 tablespoon hemp hearts
70g fresh seasonal berries

Lunch:
Turkey stir-fry made with 115g chopped turkey breast, water chestnuts, bok choy, mangetout, parsley, drizzled with 1 tablespoon flaxseed oil

Mid- to Late Afternoon:
Metabolixir (pages 196–197)

Dinner:
115g chicken browned in 1 tablespoon ghee with ginger, leeks, and broccoli
80g cooked basmati rice drizzled with 1 tablespoon pine nut oil

Treat:
1 Radical Chocolate Chip Cookie (pages 227–228)

WEDNESDAY

Breakfast:
Citrus Blaster (page 201)

Snack:
3 macadamia nuts
10 cherries

Lunch:
115g roasted chicken with lemon juice and garlic
90g cooked millet drizzled with 1 tablespoon hemp oil
Watercress and cucumber salad with 1 tablespoon Horseradish Vinaigrette (page
  224) topped with 1 tablespoon ground toasted flaxseeds

Mid- to Late Afternoon:
Metabolixir (pages 196–197)

Dinner:
1 (115g) lamb burger with mint drizzled with 1 tablespoon hemp oil
240ml Creamy Dreamy Watercress Soup (pages 218–219)

Treat:
2 squares dark chocolate and 7 almonds

THURSDAY

Breakfast:
Citrus Blaster (page 201)

Snack:
1 (single-serving) package roasted seaweed snacks
12 grapes

Lunch:

1 Radical Turkey Burger (page 207)

Salad of shredded red and green cabbage, jicama (yam beans) or cucumber, and carrots, with 1 tablespoon Sixy Sesame Salad Dressing (page 221) and sprinkled with 1 tablespoon chia seeds

80g peas with 1 tablespoon butter or ghee

Mid- to Late Afternoon:

Metabolixir (pages 196–197)

Dinner:

115g grilled lamb chops with rosemary, garlic, and pinch of cinnamon

Mashed steamed cauliflower with fennel sprinkled with 1 tablespoon ground toasted flaxseeds

Treat:

1 Hemp Cacao Magic 6-Ball (page 227)

FRIDAY

Breakfast:

Citrus Blaster (page 201)

Snack:

Veggie sticks with Sunflower "Cheese" Dip (page 224)

Lunch:

1 (115g) beef patty, drizzled with 1 tablespoon flaxseed oil

Grapefruit Slaw (page 214)

Mid- to Late Afternoon:

Metabolixir (pages 196–197)

Dinner:

Roasted Sesame Pecan Chicken (pages 209–210)

85g Roasted Beetroots with Sour Cream and Dill (page 215)

Treat:

7 almonds

SATURDAY

Breakfast:
Citrus Blaster (page 201)

Snack:
100g cottage cheese with 80g pineapple

Lunch:
115g minced turkey cooked in 1 tablespoon ghee with garlic, wrapped in
  lettuce leaves
Steamed broccoli with lemon juice and 1 tablespoon hemp hearts
Endive and cucumber salad with 1 tablespoon Horseradish Vinaigrette (page 224)

Mid- to Late Afternoon:
Metabolixir (pages 196–197)

Dinner:
115g prawns sautéed in 1 tablespoon ghee with ginger and garlic, with
  steamed broccoli
80g cooked basmati rice drizzled with 1 tablespoon of pine nut oil

Treat:
2 squares of bitter dark chocolate

WEEK 3: 21-DAY RADICAL REBOOT

SUNDAY

Breakfast:
Citrus Blaster (page 201)

Snack:
7 almonds
½ papaya drizzled with lime juice

Lunch:

85g shredded crab with celery sticks and lime juice

240ml Creamy Dreamy Watercress Soup (pages 218–219)

Mid- to Late Afternoon:

Metabolixir (pages 196–197)

Dinner:

Gingered Steaks with Rocket and Cucumber Salad (page 208) topped with 1 tablespoon hemp hearts

100g baked butternut squash with ground coriander drizzled with 1 tablespoon
flaxseed oil

Treat:

2 tablespoons pine nuts

MONDAY

Breakfast:

Citrus Blaster (page 201)

Snack:

1 (serving-size) package roasted seaweed snacks

1 small orange or tangerine

Lunch:

Radical Turkey Burger (page 207)

Salad of shredded red and green cabbage, jicama (yam beans) or cucumber, and
carrot with 1 tablespoon Sixy Sesame Salad Dressing (page 221)

80g peas with 1 tablespoon butter

Mid- to Late Afternoon:

Metabolixir (pages 196–197)

Dinner:

Savory Rosemary Lemon Lamb Chops (pages 211–212)

Mixed lettuce salad with bitter greens, sprinkled with 1 tablespoon hemp hearts and drizzled with 1 tablespoon Hempseed Vinaigrette (page 222)

80g steamed broccoli and cauliflower

Treat:

6 Crazy Good Curried Cashews (page 226)

TUESDAY

Breakfast:

Citrus Blaster (page 201)

Snack:

Cucumber spears with lime juice

1 kiwi

Lunch:

1 (115g) beef burger with mustard wrapped in romaine lettuce

85g sweet potato fries

Steamed yellow squash medley with 1 tablespoon butter or ghee, sprinkled with 1 tablespoon ground toasted flaxseeds

Mid- to Late Afternoon:

Metabolixir (pages 196–197)

Dinner:

Roasted Sesame Pecan Chicken (pages 209–210)

Oven-roasted Brussels sprouts with lemon zest, drizzled with 1 tablespoon pine nut oil

Treat:

7 almonds

WEDNESDAY

Breakfast:
Citrus Blaster (page 201)

Snack:
2 tablespoons pumpkin seeds
½ small banana

Lunch:
115g grilled chicken with capers on a bed of mixed greens, shredded daikon radish (mooli), 8 olives, drizzled with 1 tablespoon Sixy Sesame Salad Dressing (page 221) and 1 tablespoon ground toasted flaxseeds

Mid- to Late Afternoon:
Metabolixir (pages 196–197)

Dinner:
1 (115g) lamb burger with fresh mint and dill
Rocket and frisée with 1 tablespoon Hempseed Vinaigrette (page 222)
80g cooked basmati rice with 1 tablespoon butter or ghee

Treat:
2 squares bitter dark chocolate

THURSDAY

Breakfast:
Citrus Blaster (page 201)
70g fresh seasonal berries

Snack:
Pickle spears and 3 macadamia nuts

Lunch:
240ml Radical Lentil Soup (page 220)
Salad of mixed greens, grated carrot, and daikon (mooli) with 1 tablespoon Sixy
  Sesame Salad Dressing (page 221)

Mid- to Late Afternoon:
Metabolixir (pages 196–197)

Dinner:
115g grilled wild-caught salmon drizzled with 1 tablespoon hemp oil, coconut
  aminos, lemon juice, and ginger
Grapefruit Slaw (page 214)
Steamed broccolini (rapini/cime di rapa) drizzled with 1 tablespoon flaxseed oil

Treat:
4 walnuts and 2 squares dark chocolate

FRIDAY

Breakfast:
Citrus Blaster (page 201)

Snack:
Celery sticks with 2 tablespoons cashew butter and 1 tablespoon chia seeds
1 medium peach

Lunch:
115g grilled chicken breast with tarragon on bed of endive, 8 olives, daikon
  (mooli), and 1 tablespoon Umeboshi Plum Vinaigrette (page 223)
90g cooked millet with 1 tablespoon butter or ghee

Mid- to Late Afternoon:
Metabolixir (pages 196–197)

Dinner:
Grilled Lemon Dijon Turkey (pages 210–211)
Steamed green beans drizzled with lemon zest and 1 tablespoon flaxseed oil

Treat:
1 Hemp Cacao Magic 6-Ball (page 227)

SATURDAY

Breakfast:
Citrus Blaster (page 201)

Snack:
2 Brazil nuts
1 small apple

Lunch:
Chicken bowl made with 115g shredded grilled chicken, chopped celery, 8 olives, topped with 1 tablespoon Sixy Sesame Salad Dressing (page 221) and 1 tablespoon hemp hearts

Mid- to Late Afternoon:
Metabolixir (pages 196–197)

Dinner:
1 (115g) grilled steak with rosemary, drizzled with 1 tablespoon flaxseed oil
Cabbage sautéed in Bone Broth (page 216) with chopped garlic
80g peas with mint

Treat:
1 Radical Chocolate Chip Cookie (pages 227–228)

WEEK 4: MAINTENANCE PLAN

SUNDAY

Breakfast:
Citrus Blaster (page 201)

Snack:
Apple with 2 tablespoons nut butter

Lunch:
Tuna salad made with 115g tuna fish, 1 tablespoon avocado oil mayonnaise,
  chopped celery, and a pinch of curry powder
240ml Creamy Dreamy Watercress Soup (pages 218–219) topped with 1 tablespoon hemp hearts
85g steamed swede with dill drizzled with 1 tablespoon pine nut oil

Mid- to Late Afternoon:
Metabolixir (pages 196–197)

Dinner:
115g grilled chicken with lemon zest and garlic
80g steamed red cabbage with caraway seeds
80g cooked basmati rice with 1 tablespoon butter or ghee

Treat:
15 pistachios
10 cherries

MONDAY

Breakfast:
Citrus Blaster (page 201)

Snack:
1 sliced kiwi and ½ small banana, sliced

Lunch:

Curried Cauliflower Soup (pages 219–220)

Spinach and radicchio salad with Umeboshi Plum Vinaigrette (page 223)

100g baked yam or sweet potato topped with 2 chopped macadamia nuts and 1
tablespoon shredded coconut

Mid- to Late Afternoon:

Metabolixir (pages 196–197)

Dinner:

1 (115g) bison or beef burger

Steamed broccoli sprinkled with 1 tablespoon hemp hearts

90g cooked millet with 1 tablespoon butter or ghee

Treat:

1 serving Surprise! Cake (pages 228–229)

TUESDAY

Breakfast:

Citrus Blaster (page 201)

Snack:

70g mixed fresh berries topped with 1 tablespoon cream

Lunch:

115g turkey medallions with spring onions, drizzled with 1 tablespoon pine nut oil

Butterhead lettuce and shredded carrot salad with Umeboshi Plum Vinaigrette
(page 223)

Mid- to Late Afternoon:

Metabolixir (pages 196–197)

Dinner:

115g grilled lamb chops

80g mixed peas and basmati rice with mint, drizzled with olive oil

Treat:

2 squares bitter dark chocolate and 7 almonds
1 medium peach

WEDNESDAY

Breakfast:

Citrus Blaster (page 201)

Snack:

6 Crazy Good Curried Cashews (page 226)
1 small apple

Lunch:

115g prawns with shredded cabbage and 1 tablespoon Coriander Lime Dressing
  (pages 222–223)
90g cooked millet with ginger

Mid- to Late Afternoon:

Metabolixir (pages 196–197)

Dinner:

240ml Radical Lentil Soup (page 220) sprinkled with 1 tablespoon ground toasted
  flaxseeds
90g sautéed spinach with 1 tablespoon olive oil and sea salt

Treat:

1 Crunchy Almond Fruit Bar (page 229)

THURSDAY

Breakfast:

Citrus Blaster (page 201)

Snack:

Carrot sticks with 2 tablespoons cashew butter
80g mango

Lunch:

Chicken Schnitzel with Cucumber Salad (pages 206–207) sprinkled with 1 tablespoon hemp hearts

100g peeled and chopped jicama (yam beans) or cucumber drizzled with lime juice

80g cooked basmati rice drizzled with 1 tablespoon butter or ghee

Mid- to Late Afternoon:

Metabolixir (pages 196–197)

Dinner:

1 (115g) roasted turkey breast with sage and rosemary, drizzled in 1 tablespoon
extra-virgin olive oil

100g acorn squash medallions, braised in Bone Broth (page 216)

Treat:

4 walnut halves

2 medium apricots

2 squares dark chocolate

FRIDAY

Breakfast:

Citrus Blaster (page 201)

70g fresh seasonal berries

Snack:

Hummus with cucumbers and carrots

Lunch:

115g roast beef with pickles and mustard

Spinach and frisée salad with 1 tablespoon toasted flaxseeds and 1 tablespoon Sixy
Sesame Salad Dressing (page 221)

Mid- to Late Afternoon:

Metabolixir (pages 196–197)

Dinner:
Cauliflower Crust Pizza (page 213) smeared with 1 tablespoon olive oil, topped
with 115g organic minced turkey, 30g cheese, 8 black olives, artichoke hearts,
spinach, oregano, and basil
100g oven-roasted sweet potato

Treat:
1 Crunchy Almond Fruit Bar (page 229)

SATURDAY

Breakfast:
Citrus Blaster (page 201)

Snack:
2 plums

Lunch:
Teriyaki Tempeh (page 212)
Mixed green salad with ½ small avocado and 1 tablespoon Coriander Lime Dressing (pages 222–223)
90g cooked millet drizzled with 1 tablespoon butter or ghee

Mid- to Late Afternoon:
Metabolixir (pages 196–197)

Dinner:
1 (115g) Salisbury steak with coconut aminos
100g mashed sweet potato with coconut milk and cinnamon
Green leafy salad with bitter greens and 1 tablespoon Ginger Vinaigrette (page 222)

Treat:
1 slice Coconut Buttermilk Pie (page 230)

11 RADICAL RECIPES

Note: Recipes flagged with an **M** should be used only for Maintenance; all the rest are for 21-Day or Maintenance.

METABOLIXIRS
Pick-Me-Up Metabolixir
Cider Fixer Metabolixir
Dandy-as-Candy Metabolixir

JUICES & BEVERAGES
AM Rise and Shine Juice
PM High Five Juice
Radical Lemon Cubes
Val's Horchata

BREAKFASTS
Citrus Blaster
Tempeh-Basil Breakfast Scramble
Blueberry Lemon Almond Pancakes **M**
Melissa's Turkey Sausage Patties

MAIN DISHES
Gingery Asian Lettuce Wraps
Turkey Lettuce Wraps
Pineapple Prawns with Ginger
Chicken Schnitzel with Cucumber Salad
Radical Turkey Burgers
Gingered Steaks with Rocket and Cucumber Salad
Moroccan Chicken
Roasted Sesame Pecan Chicken
Grilled Lemon Dijon Turkey
Lemon Garlic Roasted Chicken
Savory Rosemary Lemon Lamb Chops

Teriyaki Tempeh
Cauliflower Crust Pizza

VEGETABLES & SIDES
Grapefruit Slaw
Roasted Beetroots with Sour Cream and Dill

SOUPS & BROTHS
Basic Bone Broth
Broth-elixirs:
> The Enchantress Broth-elixir
> Sassy Samurai Broth-elixir
> Golden Power Broth-elixir
Creamy Dreamy Watercress Soup
Curried Cauliflower Soup **M**
Radical Lentil Soup

DRESSINGS, DIPS & SAUCES
Sixy Sesame Salad Dressing
Basic Vinaigrette
> Variations:
> Greek Vinaigrette
> Dill Pickle Vinaigrette
> Miso Vinaigrette
> French-Style Vinaigrette
> Spicy Sesame Vinaigrette
> Kimchi Vinaigrette
> Ginger Vinaigrette
Hempseed Vinaigrette
Coriander Lime Dressing
Umeboshi Plum Vinaigrette
Horseradish Vinaigrette
Sunflower "Cheese" Dip
Chimichurri Sauce

SNACKS & TREATS

Crazy Good Curried Cashews

Hemp Cacao Magic 6-Balls

Radical Chocolate Chip Cookies

Surprise! Cake **M**

Crunchy Almond Fruit Bars **M**

Coconut Buttermilk Pie **M**

Almond Flour Piecrust **M**

METABOLIXIRS

On the 21-Day Reboot, you will incorporate one Metabolixir each afternoon to supercharge your digestion and metabolism. You can have them more often as desired. To maximize the benefits of the bitters (see page 54), take them thirty minutes before meals, and after meals if indigestion arises.

Pick-Me-Up Metabolixir

This lovely aperitif is a great pick-me-up before dinner. When you make your morning coffee, reserve 30ml for the Pick-Me-Up. It also makes a yummy after-dinner digestif.

Serves 1

30ml (2 tablespoons) brewed coffee

¼ teaspoon bitters

¼ teaspoon unsweetened cocoa or cacao powder

A pinch of orange zest (optional)

Stir together and enjoy!

Cider Fixer Metabolixir

This is a great aperitif if you want to get your apple cider vinegar and bitters down in one gulp.

Serves 1

60ml filtered water
1 tablespoon apple cider vinegar
¼ teaspoon bitters
¼ teaspoon ground ginger
⅛ teaspoon cayenne pepper
⅛ teaspoon yacón syrup or pure maple syrup, or 1 drop of liquid
    stevia

Stir together and enjoy!

Dandy-as-Candy Metabolixir

This delicious aperitif suits the sweeter crowd. Just don't overdo the sweet-ener—remember that you must actually *taste the bitters* for them to stimulate those digestive juices.

Serves 1

30ml (2 tablespoons) brewed roasted dandelion root tea
¼ teaspoon bitters
¼ teaspoon ground ginger
⅛ teaspoon yacón syrup or pure maple syrup, or 1 drop of liquid
    stevia
A pinch of cayenne pepper

Stir together and enjoy!

JUICES & BEVERAGES

AM Rise and Shine Juice
Makes 1 approximately 240ml serving

This antioxidant-loaded juice has turmeric to reduce inflammation, grapefruit to boost your vitamin C, and cucumber to flush out toxins—a delicious way to start your day!

- ½ grapefruit, peeled (see notes)
- 1 carrot
- 1 cucumber
- ¼ head butterhead or romaine lettuce
- 1 large handful of fresh mint leaves and stems
- 1 (2.5-cm) piece fresh ginger
- 1 (5-cm) piece fresh turmeric, or 1 teaspoon ground turmeric (see notes)
- 1 Radical Lemon Cube (page 199), thawed, or ½ lemon with peel

Clean the fruits and veggies. Process all the ingredients through a juicer or in a high-powered blender (see notes). Drink immediately for maximum nutritional benefit.

Notes: If you're on medications where grapefruit is contraindicated, you can substitute one whole orange, peeled.

If using ground turmeric, stir in at the end.

If using a high-powered blender, add enough water for a blendable consistency.

PM High Five Juice
Makes 1 approximately 240ml serving

Jicama (yam bean) is loaded with immune system-boosting nutrition, including vitamin C, magnesium, potassium, and manganese. Lemon and ginger give it pure tangy goodness with a hint of spice.

100g jicama (yam bean), peeled and roughly chopped
½ cucumber
½ apple, cored to remove seeds, peel intact
3 celery stalks
1 (5-cm) piece fresh ginger
1 Radical Lemon Cube (below), thawed, or ½ lemon with peel

Clean the fruits and veggies. Process all the ingredients through a juicer or in a high-powered blender (see note). Drink immediately for maximum nutritional benefits.

Note: If using a high-powered blender, add enough water for a blendable consistency.

Radical Lemon Cubes
Makes 24 standard-size cubes (8 cubes per lemon; 1 cube equals ⅛ whole lemon)

When life gives you lemons, make radical lemon cubes! These zesty cubes will quickly become a new household staple. When you utilize the entire lemon, you get all the phytonutrients and aromatic oils contained in the fruit. All you need is a blender and an ice cube tray. The recipe also works with limes, or a combination of lemons and limes. Use a cube any time a recipe calls for lemon juice or lemon zest, if the recipe can tolerate a little extra moisture. Add to smoothies, blended juices, or soups, or zest up a glass of water or tea.

3 lemons, quartered
240ml filtered water

Place the lemons and water in a blender or food processor and purée. Spoon the purée into ice cube trays and freeze. When frozen, the lemon cubes can be stored in a lidded container in the freezer.

Val's Horchata
Makes about 1 litre

A radical twist on a creamy, yummy classic called *kunna aya*, or Nigerian-style tigernut milk (adapted from *Nourished Kitchen* by Jennifer McGruther).

150g raw organic tigernuts
½ to 1 stick Ceylon cinnamon
1 litre warm filtered water
2 cardamom pods

Place the tigernuts and cinnamon stick in a medium-size bowl and cover with the warm filtered water. Allow to soak for 12 to 24 hours.

Combine the tigernuts, their soaking water, and the spices in a high-powered blender. Blend well until smooth, adding more cold water if necessary to facilitate even blending.

Pour the mixture into a nut milk bag and slowly press through until the solids are relatively dry, just as with making other nut milks.

The milk may be a bit too thick for your liking, so add enough filtered water to achieve a drinkable consistency.

Store the tigernut milk in a glass jar or wide-mouth jug in your refrigerator. The finer solids will settle to the bottom, in a mass, so you'll want a container that will allow you to get a spoon down into the bottom after it settles. Stirring these solids back in requires some elbow grease, but you don't want to *lose* them—they have so much of the valuable resistant fiber. Trust me . . . just shaking the jar won't do it.

Note: Horchata is wonderful over ice, or simply blended with a banana. It's also good in chia pudding, over granola, or in coffee or tea . . . it puts coconut and almond milk to shame!

BREAKFASTS

Citrus Blaster
Makes 1 approximately 240ml serving

A fat-melting, energizing boost to quick-start your weight loss.

    240ml brewed organic coffee* or roasted dandelion root tea or
        oolong tea
    1 scoop whey protein (vanilla or chocolate)
    2 tablespoons cacao powder
    2 tablespoons coconut milk
    ⅛ teaspoon ground ginger
    ¼ teaspoon ground cinnamon (Ceylon)
    ½ teaspoon powdered citrus peel (see note)
    Pinch of sea salt
    Optional: ½ teaspoon coconut sugar or a few drops of liquid stevia

Whisk all the ingredients in a small bowl or shake in a lidded jar. Pour into
your favorite glass and enjoy!

*If you don't tolerate coffee, you may use roasted dandelion root tea or oolong tea,
but realize that coffee is the absolute best for accelerating weight loss. Oolong has
50 to 75 mg of caffeine per cup, whereas coffee averages 180 mg. Dandy tea contains no caffeine. The teas may still work, but coffee is best.*

Note: Courtesy of Doc Shillington, you can make your own vitamin C complex
loaded with rutin, hesperidin, and bioflavonoids. Here's how: Save your organic
orange and lemon peels and cut into strips. Lay them out on a plate for a few days
until dry and crisp (or use a food dehydrator). Using a coffee grinder, grind peels
into a powder.

Tempeh-Basil Breakfast Scramble
Serves 2

You'll be surprised at how such a simple scramble can be so nutritious—and delicious! If you can't find watercress, try rocket.

    2 garlic cloves, finely chopped
    1 handful watercress
    2 tablespoons bone broth (see page 216 for homemade)
    1 large handful fresh basil, chopped
    450g tempeh, crumbled
    ½ teaspoon coconut aminos
    1 teaspoon freshly squeezed lemon juice

Sauté the garlic and watercress in the bone broth in a frying pan until softened.

Lower the heat to medium-low and add the basil, tempeh, coconut aminos, and lemon juice.

Cover and cook for 5 to 7 minutes, stirring occasionally.

Blueberry Lemon Almond Pancakes
Makes about 10 small pancakes

Using almond flour rather than wheat flour, these gluten-free goodies are delicately flavored but have a protein punch.

    100g almond flour
    ½ teaspoon bicarbonate of soda
    Pinch of sea salt
    1 large egg
    1 large egg white
    1 Radical Lemon Cube (page 199), thawed
    60ml filtered water, or as needed
    75g blueberries

Preheat a griddle or large frying pan to 190°C/375°F.

Stir together the almond flour, bicarbonate of soda, and salt in a bowl.

Whisk the egg, egg white, and thawed lemon cube together in a separate bowl.

Stir the flour mixture into the egg mixture, adding enough water to reach a pancake batter consistency.

Gently fold in the blueberries.

Drop the batter by large spoonfuls onto the prepared griddle and cook until the bottom of the pancakes are golden brown and the edges are dry, 3 to 4 minutes.

Flip and cook until browned on the other side, 2 to 3 minutes.

Repeat with remaining batter.

Melissa's Turkey Sausage Patties
Serves 3 to 4

Although I've put this recipe with the breakfast items, these lean, flavorful patties are perfect for any meal.

450g lean, organic minced turkey
2–6 garlic cloves, crushed
½ teaspoon rubbed sage
½ teaspoon ground fennel seeds
Sea salt

Preheat the oven to 180°C/350°F/gas 4.

Mix together all the ingredients, except the salt, in a bowl, shape the mixture into 5-cm-diameter sausage patties, and place on a grill pan or on a wire rack above a baking pan.

Bake until no pink remains in the center, 20 to 25 minutes.

Add additional sea salt to taste at the table, if necessary.

MAIN DISHES

Gingery Asian Lettuce Wraps
Makes 10 wraps

These delicately flavored wraps pack in a lot of nutrients—without the high sodium found in other wraps.

1 tablespoon ghee
550g organic pasture-raised minced beef
Sea salt
4 garlic cloves, diced
1 (2.5-cm) piece fresh ginger, diced
80g daikon radish (mooli), chopped
115g water chestnuts, rinsed, drained, and chopped
5 tablespoons all-natural, no-sugar-added almond butter
1 tablespoon coconut aminos, plus more for serving
Butterhead lettuce leaves
Optional toppings: shredded carrot, toasted sesame seeds

Heat 1 tablespoon ghee in a large frying pan.

Brown the minced beef in the frying pan and season with sea salt to taste. Transfer to a plate and set aside.

In the same pan, cook the garlic and ginger for 2 minutes.

Add the meat back to the pan along with the daikon, and water chestnuts.

Stir in the almond butter and coconut aminos and sauté everything together for a few minutes.

To serve, place the meat mixture in lettuce leaf cups and top with shredded carrot, peanuts, sesame seeds, and extra coconut aminos.

Turkey Lettuce Wraps
Serves 6

Looking for a snack, lunch, or main course? These wraps are great for any meal (especially a pack-and-go lunch)!

1 tablespoon bone broth (see page 216 for homemade)
550g lean, organic minced turkey
1 garlic clove, finely chopped
⅛ teaspoon ground ginger
100g peeled and diced jicama (yam bean) or water chestnuts
2 tablespoons coconut aminos
1 tablespoon umeboshi plum vinegar
⅛ teaspoon sea salt
12 butterhead lettuce leaves

Heat the bone broth in a large frying pan over medium-high heat.

Add the turkey, garlic, and ginger and cook, stirring occasionally, for about 6 minutes, or until the turkey is browned.

Combine the turkey mixture and jicama or water chestnuts in a large bowl, stirring well, and set aside.

Meanwhile, in a small bowl, whisk together the coconut aminos, plum vinegar, and sea salt and drizzle over the turkey mixture. Toss to coat completely.

Add about 4 tablespoons of the turkey mixture to each lettuce leaf, serve, and enjoy.

Pineapple Prawns with Ginger
Serves 4

Serve this tropical dish over basmati rice, topped with a sprinkle of coconut, for a delicious trip to the islands.

120ml bone broth (see page 216 for homemade)
1 garlic clove, finely chopped
450g shelled and deveined prawns

2 small carrots, chopped

50g chopped endive (escarole or chicory)

Sea salt

1 teaspoon ground ginger

1 teaspoon freshly grated lime zest

4 tablespoons chopped fresh coriander

80g diced fresh pineapple

Heat 2 tablespoons of the bone broth in a large frying pan over medium heat.

Add the garlic, prawns, carrots, and endive. Cook for 5 minutes, or until fragrant.

Whisk together the remaining ingredients, including the remaining 6 tablespoons of bone broth, in a medium-size bowl and pour over the prawn mixture.

Lower the heat to low and simmer for 5 to 10 minutes, or until the prawns are opaque and the vegetables are tender.

Serve warm.

Chicken Schnitzel with Cucumber Salad
Serves 4

This version of the Austrian classic has all of the crunch—and none of the unhealthy ingredients.

6 English cucumbers, sliced 1cm thick

1 teaspoon sea salt, plus more to season chicken

4 tablespoons finely chopped fresh dill, plus small sprigs for garnish

400g Greek yogurt

200g almonds, finely chopped

4 organic, pasture-raised chicken breasts, cut on the bias into 12
    thin slices, about 5mm thick

1 tablespoon ghee, for frying

In a colander, toss the cucumbers with 1 teaspoon of salt. Let stand for 15 minutes, then gently squeeze out the excess water.

Mix together the cucumbers, chopped dill, and 4 tablespoons of the yogurt in a large bowl.

Place the remaining yogurt in a shallow bowl, and the almonds in a separate shallow bowl.

Season the chicken with salt and dip into the yogurt, letting the excess drip back into the bowl. Then, dredge the chicken in the almonds, pressing to flatten the chicken and help the nuts adhere.

Heat 1 tablespoon of ghee in a large frying pan over medium-high heat until shimmering.

In batches, add the chicken to the pan in a single layer and cook over moderately high heat (adding more ghee if necessary), turning once, until browned and crispy, for about 5 minutes. Transfer to paper towels to drain.

Serve the chicken with the cucumber salad and garnish with small sprigs of dill.

Radical Turkey Burgers
Serves 4

These delicately flavored burgers are sure to be a barbecue hit!

450g lean, organic minced turkey
1 teaspoon garlic powder
1 teaspoon freshly grated lemon zest
1 teaspoon ground cumin
½ teaspoon sea salt
1 tablespoon fresh parsley, chopped

Preheat the oven to 200°C/400°F/gas 6.

Mix together the turkey, garlic powder, lemon zest, cumin, salt, and parsley in a bowl.

Shape into four equal-size patties.

Place on a baking sheet and bake for 20 to 25 minutes.

Gingered Steaks with Rocket and Cucumber Salad
Serves 4

Spices and peppery rocket take the average steak salad up a few notches.

4 medium-size beef steaks
1 tablespoon bone broth (see page 216 for homemade)
4 tablespoons coconut aminos
2 Radical Lemon Cubes (page 199), thawed
1 tablespoon freshly grated ginger
2 garlic cloves, finely chopped, plus 1 clove left whole but peeled
Sea salt
80g rocket
1 large cucumber, diced
30g chopped carrot
½ very ripe avocado, peeled and mashed
4 tablespoons freshly squeezed lime juice
2 tablespoons chopped fresh basil
1 tablespoon chopped fresh parsley

Place the steaks in a large bowl.

Whisk together the bone broth, coconut aminos, thawed lemon cubes, ginger, chopped garlic, and salt in a small bowl.

Pour the broth mixture over the steaks and cover. Refrigerate for at least 2 hours to marinate.

Heat a grill to medium heat.

Place the steaks on the grill and cook for 5 minutes on each side, or until the steaks reach your desired level of doneness. Remove from the grill, allow the steaks to cool, then slice.

Toss the sliced steak with the rocket, cucumber, and carrot in a large bowl.

Place the whole garlic clove, avocado, lime juice, and herbs in a blender and blend until smooth.

Pour the dressing over the salad, toss, and serve.

Moroccan Chicken
Serves 4 to 6

Turmeric, ginger, and cumin not only enhance the nutritional benefits of this dish, they also take you on an exotic adventure.

1.8kg organic, pasture-raised chicken legs and thighs
3 tablespoons bone broth (see page 216 for homemade)
8 Radical Lemon Cubes (page 199), thawed
2 teaspoons sea salt
1 teaspoon ground turmeric
1 tablespoon ground ginger
2 teaspoons ground cumin
1 teaspoon dried oregano

Place the chicken in a large bowl.

Pour in the bone broth, add the thawed lemon cubes, and toss to coat.

Mix the remaining ingredients together in a small bowl until well combined.

Sprinkle over the chicken, making sure to coat it evenly.

Cover, place in the refrigerator, and allow to marinate for 6 hours or overnight (longer is better).

Grill the chicken until cooked through, about 30 minutes.

Roasted Sesame Pecan Chicken
Serves 8

This simple and delicious chicken dish pairs wonderfully with a small salad.

Cooking spray
60ml almond milk or hemp milk
55g almond flour
55g finely chopped pecans
2 tablespoons sesame seeds
½ teaspoon paprika
1 teaspoon salt

8 (115g each) organic, pasture-raised boneless, skinless chicken
    breast halves, partially flattened

2 tablespoons ghee

Preheat the oven to 180°C/350°F/gas 4. Coat a 38 x 25 x 2.5cm baking tin with cooking spray.

Place the almond or hemp milk in a shallow bowl.

In another shallow bowl, combine the almond flour, chopped pecans, sesame seeds, paprika, and salt.

Dip the chicken into the milk, then coat with the almond flour mixture.

In a large, non-stick frying pan, brown the chicken in the ghee on both sides.

Transfer to the prepared baking pan.

Roast, uncovered, in the oven for 15 to 20 minutes, or until no longer pink.

Grilled Lemon Dijon Turkey
Serves 4

Herbs, lemon, and mustard create layers of flavors—and a little kick—in this turkey dish.

4 organic turkey breast strips

2 tablespoons coconut aminos

2 Radical Lemon Cubes (page 199), thawed

2 tablespoons Dijon mustard

1 teaspoon garlic powder

1 tablespoon chopped fresh sage

1 tablespoon chopped fresh rosemary

1 tablespoon chopped fresh thyme

2 tablespoons apple cider vinegar

2 tablespoons bone broth (see page 216 for homemade)

Place the turkey in a bowl.

Mix together the coconut aminos, thawed lemon cubes, mustard, garlic powder, sage, rosemary, thyme, vinegar, and bone broth in a small bowl. Pour over the turkey.

Marinate in the fridge overnight, or for at least 2 hours.

Cook on a heated grill for 4 minutes per side, or until cooked through.

Lemon Garlic Roasted Chicken
Serves 4 to 6

When the aroma of roasting garlic and chicken begin wafting through your home, no one will believe you're cooking "diet food"!

1 whole organic, pasture-raised chicken
1 tablespoon ghee, melted
Sea salt
1 lemon, zested and quartered
3 celery stalks, chopped
3 garlic cloves, smashed
2 carrots, chopped
2 tablespoons fresh rosemary

Preheat the oven to 180°C/350°F/gas 4.

Rub the chicken all over with the ghee, including the inside cavity, and sprinkle with the sea salt and lemon zest. Stuff the cavity with the lemon quarters, chopped celery, garlic, chopped carrot, and 1 tablespoon of the rosemary. Sprinkle the outside of the chicken with the remaining tablespoon of rosemary.

Roast, uncovered, in the oven for 1½ hours, or until a meat thermometer reads 74°C/165°F.

Savory Rosemary Lemon Lamb Chops
Serves 2

Whether it's Easter or just another Sunday, this lamb dish is both simple and savory.

2 tablespoons ghee, at room temperature
4 Radical Lemon Cubes (page 199), thawed
4 lamb chops

1 teaspoon garlic powder
1 teaspoon sea salt
1 tablespoon dried rosemary

Preheat the oven to 180°C/350°F/gas 4.

Whisk the ghee and thawed lemon cubes together in a small bowl.

Using a pastry brush, coat each side of the lamb chops with the ghee mixture. Sprinkle each chop on both sides with garlic powder, sea salt, and dried rosemary.

Bake on a baking sheet for 20 to 30 minutes, or until the lamb reaches your desired doneness.

Teriyaki Tempeh
Serves 2

Teriyaki is the perfect complement to the nutty taste of tempeh. Serve with cooked millet for a protein-hearty meal.

2 tablespoons ghee
1 (225g) package tempeh, cut into 1-cm strips
1 teaspoon garlic powder
2 tablespoons coconut aminos
1 tablespoon chopped almonds
¼ head red cabbage, shredded
2 carrots, sliced diagonally into ovals
1 (225g) can sliced water chestnuts, rinsed and drained
1 (225g) can bamboo shoots, rinsed and drained

Preheat the oven to 230°C/450°F/gas 8. Rub the ghee on the bottom and sides of an ovenproof, lidded pan.

Sprinkle the tempeh with the garlic powder and place it in the prepared pan.

Mix together the coconut aminos and almonds in a small bowl to make a teriyaki sauce.

Spoon half of the mixture over the tempeh.

Add the cabbage, carrots, water chestnuts, and bamboo shoots in layers.

Pour the rest of the sauce over all.

Cover and bake for 45 minutes.

Cauliflower Crust Pizza
Makes 1 23cm pizza

You heard it here: Cauliflower is "the new kale." Try it as pizza crust and you'll never go back to dough again! This recipe can be easily doubled.

1 tablespoon unsalted butter or ghee
115g cauliflower
1 large egg
50g Parmesan cheese, grated
1 teaspoon Italian seasoning
½ teaspoon finely chopped garlic
Toppings, such as mozzarella, tomato, artichoke, spinach, rocket,
        minced beef, chicken, etc.

Preheat the oven to 230°C/450°F/gas 8. Line a baking sheet with parchment paper and grease lightly with the butter.

Pulse the cauliflower in a food processor until it has a ricelike consistency, or grate with a cheese grater.

Steam the cauliflower for 3 to 5 minutes, then drain in a fine-mesh strainer, pressing gently to remove any moisture. Transfer to a clean tea towel, wrap the towel around the cauliflower, and gently press out any remaining moisture.

Combine the cauliflower, egg, cheese, Italian seasoning, and garlic in a medium-size bowl and mix well.

Transfer the cauliflower mixture to the prepared baking sheet and pat out to form a 23-cm round. Bake for 15 minutes.

Add your choice of toppings and pop under a preheated grill for just long enough to melt the cheese in the topping.

Return to the oven and roast for another 10 minutes.

VEGETABLES & SIDES

Grapefruit Slaw
Serves 4

This tangy slaw is a great summertime accompaniment to chicken and fish. If you're on medications where grapefruit is contraindicated, you can substitute oranges.

225g Chinese leaf, thinly sliced
2 pink grapefruit, peeled and segmented, 1 tablespoon juice
    reserved
1 celery stalk, thinly sliced on a diagonal
30g coarsely grated carrot
30g diced red radish
1½ tablespoons umeboshi plum vinegar
½ teaspoon finely grated lime zest
1½ teaspoons freshly squeezed lime juice
2 tablespoons pumpkin seeds
1 tablespoon coarsely chopped fresh flat-leaf parsley
Sea salt

Mix together the cabbage, grapefruit, celery, carrot, and radish in a medium-size bowl.

Whisk together the reserved grapefruit juice, plum vinegar, and lime zest and juice in a small bowl.

Toss the slaw with the dressing. Sprinkle with the pumpkin seeds, parsley, and salt to taste.

Roasted Beetroots with Sour Cream and Dill
Serves 4

Sweet, creamy, tangy, and dilly . . . what's not to love? Beetroots work wonders for digestion, blood pressure, and detoxification.

3 to 4 beetroots (remove greens for another use, such as a greens
    sauté or soup)
60ml cultured sour cream
1 tablespoon fresh dill, or 1 teaspoon dried
Sea salt

Preheat the oven to 220°C/425°F/gas 7.

Wash and trim the beetroots.

Place on a baking sheet and roast in the oven until a knife slides in easily, about 45 minutes. When cool enough to handle, slide off the beetroot skins.

Dice the beetroots and toss with the sour cream, dill, and salt to taste. Serve warm or at room temperature.

SOUPS & BROTHS

Basic Bone Broth
Makes 4 to 5 litres broth

This basic recipe is for chicken bone broth, but it can be adapted for beef or other bones. Just swap in the same amount of meat.

Chicken: 1–1.8kg pasture-raised necks/backs/feet/wings (whatever you have available). You can also use whole chicken or turkey carcasses. The point is to fill up your slow cooker with lots of bones and simmer the heck out of them. Use parts only from happy, organic, pastured birds.

Onion: 1 medium-size onion, peel on and quartered (omit for 21-Day Radical Reboot)

Garlic: 4 to 6 unpeeled garlic cloves, smashed

Bay leaves: 2

Fresh thyme: Several sprigs

Parsley: 1 bunch

Filtered water: Fill the slow cooker to its max-fill line, which will just cover the solids

Apple cider vinegar: 2 tablespoons (helps extract minerals from the bones)

Place all the solid ingredients in a 6-litre slow cooker. Add the water and vinegar.

Simmer for 24 to 48 hours on LOW to MEDIUM (depending on your slow cooker, LOW might be a little too low).

Turn off the heat and allow to cool slightly. Strain the broth through a colander into a large bowl, and discard the solids. You'll end up with 4 to 5 litres, depending on the bones-to-water ratio.

Fill wide-mouth, litre-size preserving jars with the warm broth, making sure to leave jar space for expansion during freezing. The fluid level should be no higher than the jar shoulder. It's easier to use a measuring cup than a ladle to fill them. Take care to not overtighten the lids, which will snug up in the refrigerator when the broth cools.

Immediately put the jars into the fridge. If planning to freeze the broth, allow to chill in the fridge, then transfer the jars to the freezer. Use within a week if refrigerated, or freeze for up to 3 months.

Radical Tips

A great time-saver is the Soup Sock! A Soup Sock is a disposable stretchy mesh bag (much like cheesecloth) that you can put all the solid ingredients into before placing in the slow cooker. When your broth is done, cleanup is much easier because you don't have to strain it—you just lift out the sock and put it in the garbage!

Freeze some of your bone broth in ice cube trays for easy additions into stir-fries and other dishes.

Broth-elixirs: Less Than a Soup and More Than a Beverage

Feel like something warm but not heavy . . . not a meal but something a little more substantial than tea? Introducing the Broth-elixirs! Broth drinks have become trendy foods in boutique dining establishments across the country, so we've developed three simple, tasty recipes of our own. These are quick to put together and make the perfect light lunch or bedtime snack. You can use homemade bone broth (page 216) or a good commercial organic variety.

The instructions are easy: Just stir together the ingredients in a mug and enjoy!

The Enchantress Broth-elixir
240ml warm bone broth
1 teaspoon pine nut oil
½ teaspoon umeboshi plum vinegar
½ teaspoon salt
½ teaspoon garam masala

Umeboshi plum vinegar provides a lovely, slightly salty tang, as well as adding probiotic benefits.

Sassy Samurai Broth-elixir
240ml warm bone broth
1 teaspoon pine nut oil
1 teaspoon coconut aminos
½ teaspoon ground ginger
Pinch of cayenne pepper

Ginger and cayenne are not for the faint of heart. Give your inner samurai a fat-burning boost! Cayenne pepper also helps cleanse the blood.

Golden Power Broth-elixir
240ml warm bone broth
1 teaspoon pine nut oil
½ teaspoon freshly squeezed lemon juice
½ teaspoon sea salt
¼ teaspoon ground turmeric
¼ teaspoon ground cumin
Pinch of freshly ground black pepper
Pinch of cayenne pepper

Turmeric wins the gold for beating inflammation, and just a hint of black pepper to ensure optimal absorption.

Creamy Dreamy Watercress Soup
Makes 1.5 litres

This delicious soup makes it easy for you to access all the health benefits of watercress. If watercress is not available, substitute rocket. Use celeriac, instead of cauliflower if you prefer.

1 litre bone broth (for homemade, see page 216)
½ large head cauliflower, cut into large stalks and florets
1 (5-cm) piece fresh ginger, peeled and chopped
2–3 leeks, cleaned and sliced
1 daikon radish (mooli), roughly chopped
1–2 teaspoons sea salt, to taste
1 Radical Lemon Cube (page 199)

1 large bunch watercress, roughly chopped

Optional: Add ½ to 1 teaspoon miso to each warm bowl of soup

Bring the broth to a simmer in a saucepan. Add the cauliflower, ginger, leeks, and daikon. Add enough water to the pot to just submerge the vegetables. Simmer for 20 minutes, or until the veggies are tender.

Using a handheld stick blender, blend until creamy. If too thick, you can always add a bit more water. Stir in the salt, lemon cube, watercress, and miso, if using. Simmer for 5 minutes, then blend again with your stick blender.

Serve in a mug or bowl.

Freezes well.

Curried Cauliflower Soup
Makes 4 litres

With curry, coconut, and tahini, this rich, restaurant-worthy soup delivers flavor with every mouthful. (Note: This recipe is appropriate only for the Maintenance phase, due to the coconut milk.)

1 large head cauliflower, cut into large stalks and florets

1 onion, quartered and roughly chopped

1 litre chicken bone broth (for homemade, see page 216)

750ml filtered water

2 (400ml) cans coconut milk

2 tablespoons curry powder

½ teaspoon cayenne pepper (omit if you're using a hot curry)

Sea salt

1 tablespoon tahini

Pine nut oil, for drizzling

Optional: fresh parsley or corrainder, for garnish

Combine the cauliflower, onion, bone broth, and water in a large stockpot. Bring to a gentle boil, then simmer over low-medium heat until the veggies are tender, 20 to 30 minutes. Purée, using a stick blender or regular blender. (If using a regular blender, return the mixture back to the pot after blending.)

Add the coconut milk, curry, cayenne (if using), and salt. Dissolve the tahini into a few tablespoons of the hot soup, then add to the pot and blend well—the stick blender works nicely for this. Simmer over low heat for about 20 minutes to allow the flavors to mingle.

Serve with a little drizzle of pine nut oil and garnish with fresh parsley or coriander. This soup freezes nicely in litre-size preserving jars, after cooling first in the fridge.

Radical Lentil Soup
Makes 1 litre

This protein-packed soup is a fantastic staple for lunch or dinner.

> 200g green lentils, washed and soaked overnight in 1 litre filtered water, then drained
> 750ml filtered water
> 2 tablespoons ghee
> 1 Radical Lemon Cube (page 199)
> 3 garlic cloves, chopped
> 2 celery stalks, chopped
> 1 carrot, chopped
> 2 tablespoons chopped fresh parsley
> 1 bay leaf
> ¾ teaspoon sea salt
> ½ teaspoon mustard seeds
> ½ teaspoon ground cumin

Place the drained lentils and water in a pot and cover. Bring to a boil and then lower the heat to a simmer. Add the ghee and lemon cube. Simmer for 30 minutes, or until the lentils are tender.

Add the garlic, celery, carrot, parsley, bay leaf, sea salt, mustard seeds, and cumin. Simmer, covered, for an additional 20 to 30 minutes, or until the vegetables are tender.

Freezes well.

DRESSINGS, DIPS & SAUCES

Sixy Sesame Salad Dressing
Makes 420ml

This tasty Asian-inspired dressing gives you a dose of bitters and probiotics. Although it's designed to go on a salad, I dare you not to eat it right out of the jar!

240ml dandelion root tea
70g tahini
115g cultured sour cream
3 tablespoons freshly squeezed lemon juice
1 tablespoon coconut aminos
1 garlic clove
1 (1-cm) piece fresh ginger, peeled
¼ teaspoon ground cumin
¼ teaspoon cayenne pepper
Sea salt as needed

Whiz up in a blender and you're all set!
   Store in a lidded glass jar in the fridge.

Basic Vinaigrette
Makes 240ml

This recipe may be basic, but it's a fail-safe go-to with endless variations.

3 tablespoons umeboshi plum vinegar or apple cider vinegar
1 garlic clove, finely chopped
1 teaspoon Dijon mustard
180ml olive oil (hemp oil can also be used, or a combination)
1 tablespoon finely chopped fresh herbs, or 1 teaspoon dried
Sea salt as needed

Whisk all the ingredients together in a glass bowl, or place in a glass jar and shake until thoroughly combined.

Variations: Greek Vinaigrette: Add 1 teaspoon of chopped fresh oregano and ½ teaspoon of finely grated lemon zest.

Dill Pickle Vinaigrette: Purée with 1 chopped large kosher dill pickle.

Miso Vinaigrette: Add 1 tablespoon of white miso paste.

French-Style Vinaigrette: Add 1 teaspoon of chopped fresh tarragon.

Spicy Sesame Vinaigrette: Add 1 tablespoon of toasted sesame seeds, 1 tablespoon of toasted sesame oil, and 1 teaspoon of crushed chili flakes.

Kimchi Vinaigrette: Add 2 tablespoons of finely chopped cabbage kimchi.

Ginger Vinaigrette: Add 2 tablespoons of finely chopped, peeled fresh ginger.

Hempseed Vinaigrette
Makes 240ml

Hemp's delicious nutty flavor really complements the plum vinegar here. As a bonus: You won't believe how much protein is hiding in this vinaigrette!

3 tablespoons umeboshi plum vinegar
1 garlic clove, minced
1 teaspoon Dijon mustard
180ml hemp oil
1 tablespoon hempseeds
¼ teaspoon sea salt, or to taste

Whisk all the ingredients together in a small bowl.

Coriander Lime Dressing
Makes 350ml

With its fiesta flair, this dressing is great on a salad to accompany Mexican food, or as a light snack on asparagus or sticks of carrot, celery or cucumber.

120ml bone broth (for homemade, see page 216)
4 tablespoons freshly squeezed lime juice
2 tablespoons pine nut oil
1 large handful chopped fresh coriander
¼ teaspoon sea salt
4 tablespoons (35g) sesame seeds

Combine the bone broth, lime juice, pine nut oil, coriander, and salt in a blender and process until smooth. Transfer to a small bowl.

Stir in the sesame seeds.

Umeboshi Plum Vinaigrette
Makes about 350ml

Umeboshi is a tart, salty condiment that stimulates digestion and helps to release toxins. Great on salads, but equally tasty on cooked veggies.

1–2 tablespoons umeboshi plum paste, or 2 large umeboshi plums, seeded and chopped
¼ teaspoon apple cider vinegar
4 tablespoons MCT oil
1 teaspoon sesame oil
1 teaspoon yacón syrup, coconut sugar, or a few drops of liquid stevia, to taste
2 teaspoons sesame seeds

Combine the umeboshi plum, vinegar, MCT oil, sesame oil, and sweetener in a blender and purée. Transfer to a small bowl.

Stir in the sesame seeds.

Horseradish Vinaigrette
Makes 240ml

Rev up your metabolism with this fiery flavor!

2 tablespoons prepared horseradish
2 tablespoons Dijon mustard, or 2 tablespoons dry mustard
120ml hemp oil
2 tablespoons chopped fresh parsley

Whisk all the ingredients together in a small bowl until thoroughly combined.

Sunflower "Cheese" Dip
Makes about 350ml

With the consistency of a dairy cheese dip, this easy blend is so much tastier than anything from the grocery! Delicious on fresh cut veggies, or thinned a bit for drizzling over a fresh green salad.

250g raw (hulled) sunflower seeds
2 tablespoons pine nut oil
10g fresh dill
2 tablespoons freshly squeezed lemon juice
2 garlic cloves, chopped
180ml filtered water, plus more as needed
½ teaspoon sea salt

Combine all the ingredients in a blender or food processor and pulse until combined.

Adjust the amount of water to get the consistency you like.

Chimichurri Sauce
Makes 240ml

This dressing tastes as unique as it sounds! A wonderful accompaniment to chicken, fish, or steamed vegetables. For a special treat, have it as a dipping sauce with your favorite gluten-free bread.

    2 large handfuls firmly packed flat-leaf parsley
    3–4 garlic cloves
    2 tablespoons fresh oregano leaves, or 2 teaspoons dried
    5 tablespoons extra-virgin olive oil
    2 tablespoons umeboshi plum vinegar
    ½ teaspoon sea salt

Finely chop the parsley, garlic, and oregano or gently pulse (four or five times) in a food processor. Place in a small bowl.

Stir in the remaining ingredients.

SNACKS & TREATS

Crazy Good Curried Cashews
Makes about 250g

These flavored nuts are great to take on a road trip or to work—just be sure to *hide* them from your officemates or they'll disappear in a flash!

> 250g raw cashews
> 750ml filtered water
> 1 tablespoon sea salt
> *Spice mix:*
> 2 tablespoons curry powder
> 1 teaspoon cayenne pepper
> 1 teaspoon paprika
> 1 teaspoon sea salt

Soak the cashews: Place the cashews, water, and sea salt in a bowl and stir around. Cover with a pan lid and set aside for 2 to 3 hours. Pour into a strainer set in the sink and let the nuts drain for 10 minutes.

Preheat the oven to 65°C/150°F (unless you have a food dehydrator, which is ideal). Line a baking sheet with parchment paper.

Prepare the spice mix: Mix the spices in a small bowl and toss with the cashews.

Spread the cashews evenly in a single layer on the prepared baking sheet. Slow roast in the oven for 3 to 5 hours, or follow the directions for your dehydrator. Taste occasionally. The nuts should not be moist or mushy in the middle, and they will continue to crisp as they cool.

All moisture should be gone before storing, to avoid mold problems. Allow to cool thoroughly before storing in an airtight container.

Hemp Cacao Magic 6-Balls
Makes 20–24 balls

These little balls of energy are great as a snack by themselves—and they also pair wonderfully with coffee. Note: During the 21-Day Reboot, substitute hemp oil for coconut manna.

40g raw cacao powder
150g walnuts
80g hemp hearts
4 tablespoons coconut manna (coconut butter)
1 teaspoon pure vanilla extract
1 tablespoon natural sweetener, such as pure maple syrup, or to taste
Zest of 1 orange
2 teaspoons ground cinnamon
1 teaspoon ground ginger
1 teaspoon sea salt
½ teaspoon ground cardamom
For coating: hemp hearts, cacao powder, or finely chopped walnuts

Combine all the ingredients, except the coating, in a food processor. Process until the mixture is smooth, or if you prefer, leave chunkier but processed enough to hold together when squeezed with fingers.

Form into balls and roll in additional hemp hearts, cacao powder, or ground walnuts.

Store in the fridge, or make a double batch and freeze half for later.

Radical Chocolate Chip Cookies
Makes 30 cookies

Yes, you can have cookies and have a radical metabolism! A classic treat made wholesome and delicious.

200g blanched almond flour
3–4 tablespoons coconut sugar
¼ teaspoon sea salt

½ teaspoon bicarbonate of soda

55g pastured unsalted butter

1 tablespoon pure vanilla extract

80g unsweetened carob chips

Preheat the oven to 180°C/350°F/gas 4. Line a baking sheet with parchment paper.

Combine the almond flour, coconut sugar, salt, and bicarbonate of soda in a food processor. Pulse in the butter and vanilla until a dough forms.

Remove the blade from the processor and stir in the carob chips by hand.

Scoop the dough, 1 tablespoon at a time, onto the prepared baking sheet leaving space around each spoonful, and press down gently.

Bake for 6 to 8 minutes, or until the cookies appear set and are lightly browned around the edges.

Surprise! Cake
Serves 6

This is your new go-to for all of life's celebrations. The surprise in this delicious cake is the addition of white beans, which add protein and a velvety texture to the batter. If you are a chocolate lover, see below for a chocolate variation.

360g canned organic unsalted white beans, drained and rinsed

6 large eggs

6–8 tablespoons coconut sugar

1 teaspoon pure vanilla extract

55g coconut oil, melted

50g coconut flour, sifted

½ teaspoon sea salt

1 teaspoon bicarbonate of soda

1½ teaspoons aluminum-free baking powder

Preheat the oven to 165°C/325°F/gas 3. Line a 20- to 23-cm springform tin or round cake tin with parchment paper.

Combine the beans, eggs, coconut sugar, and vanilla in a food processor.

Add the coconut oil, coconut flour, salt, bicarbonate of soda, and baking powder and purée well.

Pour the mixture into the prepared pan.

Bake for about 30 minutes. Check to see whether it's done by inserting a knife or toothpick into the middle; it's done if the tester comes out clean.

Variation: For chocolate cake, melt 40g of unsweetened organic chocolate and stir into the batter.

Crunchy Almond Fruit Bars
Makes 1 20-cm square tin

Wrap these individually for a grab-and-go bar that's actually healthy!

250g organic almond butter
60ml filtered water
3 tablespoons yacón syrup or pure maple syrup
1 teaspoon pure vanilla extract
50g shredded unsweetened coconut
80g blueberries
1 tablespoon ground chia seeds
2 teaspoons ground cinnamon
¼ teaspoon ground allspice
½ teaspoon aluminum-free baking powder
¼ teaspoon sea salt
¼ teaspoon bicarbonate of soda

Preheat the oven to 180°C/350°F/gas 4. Butter a 20-cm square baking tin.

Beat together the almond butter, water, yacón syrup, vanilla, and coconut in a large bowl, using an electric mixer.

Add the blueberries, chia seeds, cinnamon, allspice, baking powder, salt, and bicarbonate of soda and beat again until incorporated.

Pour the batter into the prepared tin and spread evenly.

Bake for about 20 minutes, or until the bars appear done.

Remove from the oven and allow to cool on a wire rack before serving. When cool, cut into bars and refrigerate or freeze.

Coconut Buttermilk Pie
Serves 6

Simply put, this pie is creamy, dreamy, and delicious.

    1 Almond Flour Piecrust dough (see below)
    3 large eggs, slightly beaten
    ½ teaspoon sea salt
    8 tablespoons buttermilk powder (or egg white protein powder)
    6–8 tablespoons coconut sugar
    480ml organic double cream, scalded (not boiled)
    1 teaspoon coconut extract
    Topping
    Whipped cream (240ml double cream, ½ teaspoon pure vanilla
        extract, plus natural sweetener such as coconut sugar to taste)
    100g toasted shredded unsweetened coconut
    1 teaspoon freshly grated nutmeg

Preheat the oven to 150°C/300°F/gas 2. Press the piecrust dough into a 23-cm pie dish, then set aside.

Combine the eggs, salt, buttermilk (or protein powder), and coconut sugar in a large bowl, and mix well.

Add the cream and coconut extract slowly, and mix well.

Pour into the piecrust. Bake for 45 to 60 minutes, or until set.

Top with whipped cream, toasted coconut, and freshly grated nutmeg.

Almond Flour Piecrust

This recipe will be passed on through the generations. Substitute it in all your favorite pie recipes. For a double crust, simply double the recipe.

Makes 1 23-cm crust

    200g blanched almond flour
    ¼ teaspoon sea salt
    2 tablespoons unsalted butter or ghee, melted
    1 large egg

Combine the almond flour and salt in a bowl. Add the butter and egg and mix until it forms a ball. Press into a 23-cm pie dish. If unfilled, bake in a preheated 180°C/350°F/gas 4 oven for 8 to 12 minutes, or until lightly browned; or bake as directed for a filled pie recipe.

ACKNOWLEDGMENTS

I am eternally grateful to my extraordinary Radical Team for their talent and ingenuity. First and foremost, to my soul sister Valerie Burke whose work ethic is the "stuff" from which legends are made. She captured my passion, my nuances, my concerns like the pro she is in every way.

Kudos to my literary agent Coleen O'Shea for her tireless efforts in being one of my Number One advocates in all things literary. My deepest thanks to Renée Sedliar who bought this book and has believed in me for over a decade. I must also acknowledge Stuart Gittleman for managing my schedule and engagements, and James Templeton and Teresa Pfaff on the home front for their TLC.

My deepest gratitude to Katie Malm for her terrific editing, and to all the folks at Da Capo Press, including editor extraordinaire Renée Sedliar, John Radziewicz, Kevin Hanover, Quinn Fariel, Mike Giarratano, Miriam Riad, and Cisca Schreefel, for helping us cross the finish line.

A heartfelt thanks to my special Beta Group for test-driving the program and sharing their valuable feedback: Catherine Vern, Marina Didenko, Carol Templeton Volanski, Lynn Tapper, Tami J. Olds Carroll, Maddy Leonard, Cheryl Riccioli, Kim Perkins Mollenkamp, Amm Ram, Bill Davis, Leslie Ashbury Farley, Ann Rhody, Nell Tate Moore, Cheryl Edwards, Debbie-Kenny Jutras, Jen Lea, Deb Heesen, Tiffany Tracy Sutphin, Sheela Hewitt, Nina Moreau, Denise McKneely Hanson, Diana Sherby, Bernice Gannuscio Zampano, Liz Beck, Kathleen Sullivan, Kim Lowe, Vicky Ganem Osollo, Suzanne Klein, Caroline Courtney, Marianne Lombardi Fogelson, Joan Strimple, and Olga Vinograd.

Finally, I bless and honor the memory of the wayshowers whose writing so inspired me: Linda Clark; Carleton Fredericks, PhD; Dr. Robert Atkins; Paavo Airola, ND; Dr. Hazel Parcells; Hanna Kroeger; Dr. Billy Crook; Dr. Orian Truss; Nathan Pritikin; Dr. Lendon Smith; Dr. Robert Mendelsohn; Dr. Nicholas Gonzalez; Gayelord Hauser; Dr. Hall Huggins; Dr. William Donald Kelley; Dr. Paul Eck; Kathryn Elwood; and Ann Wigmore.

Last but not least, a most sincere thank you to my first literary agent, Mike Cohn, who started me on my writing path, and a loving acknowledgment to the late publisher Nathan Keats.

APPENDIX 1: LIPID LINGO GLOSSARY

LIPID LINGO GLOSSARY	
Phospholipids	Complex phosphorous-containing lipid compounds that arrange themselves into dual layers, referred to as the "phospholipid bilayer." One end of the phospholipid molecule attracts water but the other end repels it. Natural phospholipids include lecithin, fat-soluble vitamins, and waxes.
Phosphatidylcholine (PC)	Class of phospholipids that contain choline, a water-soluble vitamin-like essential nutrient. PC is a major structural component of biological membranes, including cell membranes, accounting for 50 percent by weight. PC is made up of 64 percent fatty acids. Lecithin is dipalmitoyl phosphatidylcholine.
Cholesterol	Extremely important structural fat occupying 30 to 40 percent of cell membranes, by volume; precursor to hormones and bile acids; necessary for metabolizing fat soluble vitamins A, D, E, and K. In the bloodstream, cholesterol combines with fatty acids to form high-density and low-density lipoproteins (HDL and LDL); present in all parts of the body. Cholesterol is made by the body and obtained from foods.
Fatty acids	Key constituents of lipids.
Essential fatty acids (EFAs)	Fatty acids that cannot be made by the body, so they must be obtained from your foods. Omega-3 and omega-6 are the two types.
Saturated fatty acids (SFAs)	Most commonly found in animal products, saturated fats are the most stable fats because they have no double bonds in the fatty acid chain. They are nonessential to your body (not bioactive) and tend to be solid at room temperature.
Monounsaturated fatty acids (MUFAs)	Fatty acids with one double bond in the fatty acid chain; nonessential fats (not bioactive). Macadamia nut oil is highest in MUFAs (see "Omega-7"); other MUFAs include olives, avocados, peanuts, and their oils. MUFA oils are liquid at room temperature and semisolid or solid when refrigerated.
Polyunsaturated fatty acids (PUFAs)	Fatty acids with two or more double bonds in the fatty acid chain; they include omega-6 and omega-3 fatty acids.
Unsaturated fatty acids	Monounsaturated and polyunsaturated fatty acids.
Omega-6 fatty acids	Important structural elements in cell membranes and precursors to bioactive lipid mediators; energy source; involved in gene expression.
Linoleic acid (LA)	A primary PUFA and the most abundant omega-6. Primary support for cell membranes, cardiolipin, and mitochondria. Derived mostly from seeds and seed oils (raw sunflower seeds, high-linoleic sunflower oil, and high-linoleic safflower oil, nuts including pine nuts, sesame seeds). Damaged LA is found in commercial products due to heavy heating and processing, which has none of the health benefits and is destructive to cell membranes.
Arachidonic acid (AA)	A PUFA comprising 14 percent of the lipids in cell membranes and represents the largest concentration of lipid energy in the body. Described as the "CEO of the metabolic corporation"; used to make essential series 2 prostaglandins, which are your primary eicosanoids, crucial for inflammatory processes. Necessary for thought, motion, sensory perception, DNA, fetal development, and much more. Mostly animal sources (meat, butter, cream).

LIPID LINGO GLOSSARY

Gamma-linolenic acid (GLA)	A PUFA that promotes fat-burning by activating brown fat. The body converts LA into GLA and eventually into inflammatory series I prostaglandins. GLA can be converted into AA but only with difficulty. Natural sources of GLA include blackcurrant seed oil (15 percent), borage oil (not recommended), hemp seeds, and evening primrose oil.
Omega-3 fatty acids	Important structural components of cell membranes and precursors to bioactive lipid mediators. An energy source. Involved in gene expression.
Eicosapentaenoic acid (EPA)	Long-chain PUFA used primarily to make prostaglandins. Primarily marine sources.
Docosahexaenoic acid (DHA)	Long-chain PUFA used by brain, nervous system, eyes. Primarily marine sources.
Alpha-linolenic acid (ALA)	Primary PUFA building block for EPA and DHA. Approximately 85 percent of ALA is used by the body for energy. Sources include flaxseeds and flax oil, chia seeds, pumpkin seeds and oil, and perilla seed oil (54 to 64 percent).
Parent Essential Oils (PEOs)	The whole, unadulterated, and fully functional forms of omega-3 and omega-6 fatty acids (alpha-linolenic and linoleic). Top sources are nuts and seeds and their oils.
Omega-9 fatty acids (oleic acid)	Nonessential MUFA found in olives, macadamias, avocados, almonds, pecans, cashews, and other nuts. Olive oil is praised for its health benefits, but the benefits are probably the result of polyphenols in olive oil, not the MUFAs.
Omega-7 fatty acids	Another MUFA. One unique form, palmitoleic acid, has copious benefits for metabolic syndrome and heart health. Sources of palmitoleic acid include macadamia nuts, sea buckthorn, and deep sea anchovies.
Medium-chain triglycerides (MCTs)	A.k.a. medium-chain fatty acids; MCTs have 6 to 12 carbon atoms. Helpful for fat burning and stimulating metabolism. Rapidly broken down and absorbed by the body, going straight to the liver for use as energy (ketones), and not requiring bile for digestion; therefore, less likely to be stored as fat. Alternative energy source for the brain, which normally uses glucose for fuel. MCTs are found in coconut oil (60 percent), palm kernel oil (50 percent), and dairy (10–12 percent).
Cis fatty acids	Fats with biologically compatible molecular structures, rounded or bent so they help form a proper barrier in the wall of the cell membrane.
Trans fatty acids	Fats that have been "bent out of shape"—abnormally straightened—by heat and/or hydrogenation. Trans fats *transect* cell walls, increasing their permeability and leaving them open to invasion by viruses, bacteria, and foreign substances, and vulnerable to loss of essential nutrients. Trans fats from partially hydrogenated vegetable oils, such as margarine and butter substitutes, are toxic to cells and distort many of their normal physiological functions.

APPENDIX 2: RADICAL SUPPLEMENTS

If forgiveness is medicine for the soul, then gratitude is vitamins.
—Dr. Steve Maraboli

Supplements can accelerate your weight loss and enhance your overall health, especially if you have digestive issues or if you've had your gallbladder surgically removed. I have listed foundational supplements in the following table. Don't be overwhelmed when you look at the list—it's intended to be broad, with many options to enhance your success. You must evaluate which supplements are the most appropriate for you, based on your own unique set of health challenges and where your particular body needs support. Discussing your plan with a trusted health-care practitioner may be helpful.

When choosing supplements, there are a few things to keep in mind. Make certain your multivitamin-multimineral supplement is copper-free. In Chapter 7 we discussed the problems with copper overload (potential for causing estrogen dominance, thyroid issues, mood instability, and other problems). Also, be careful to check for iron content if you have iron overload issues.

SUPPLEMENTS

GALLBLADDER, BILE & LEAKY GUT

SUPPLEMENT	BENEFITS	RECOMMENDED DOSE
Bile support Choline Taurine Lipase Ox bile	Mandatory *if* no gallbladder. Highly recommended for others, especially those with gallbladder, digestion, or weight issues. Breaks down fats, thins the bile and increases bile flow, decreases fat deposition in liver, reduces homocysteine levels, precursor to acetylcholine; detoxification support	Choline: 500 mg with each meal or as directed by health-care practitioner Taurine: 250 mg with each meal or as directed by health-care practitioner Lipase: 1,500 USP 50 mg with each meal Ox bile: 100 mg per meal
Digestive bitters Metabolixirs (See Chapter 11)	Remedy for GERD, protein and fat digestion, low stomach acid	Take 30 minutes before each meal, or after a meal for digestive symptoms
Pancreatic enzymes	Breaks down proteins, fats, and carbohydrates	1–3 tablets daily with meals for digestion, or as directed by health-care practitioner
Siberian pine nut oil	Healing the digestive tract, aiding digestion and metabolism, stimulating cholecystokinin	One teaspoon 3 times daily 30–60 minutes before meals
Stomach acid replacements Hydrochloric acid (HCl), apple cider vinegar	Boosts stomach acidity, relieves acid reflux and GERD, improves fat and protein digestion, defends against gastrointestinal pathogens	Apple cider vinegar: 1 tablespoon before meals, diluted 2–3 times in water if necessary
Stoneroot (collinsonia root)	Helps dissolve gallstones, remedies constipation	1,000 to 4,000 mg per day or as directed by health-care practitioner

PROTEIN & AMINO ACIDS

MAP (Master Amino Pattern)	Protein replacement/supplement	5 tablets 3 times daily before meals (each dose equals 10 grams protein)
Protein powder	Protein replacement/supplement	20 grams of protein per serving
L-carnitine tartrate	Thermogenesis, increased energy, and mitochondrial support	1–4 grams per day in divided doses, between meals

ADRENAL, THYROID, LIVER & DETOX

Adrenal glandulars	Overall adrenal support, stress modulation, and better sleep	Dosages and blends vary, but all are typically taken 3 times per day at 7 a.m., 11 a.m., and 3 p.m., or as directed by health-care practitioner
Silver nasal spray	Antiviral, antibacterial, antifungal support for immune system	Refer to product label or as directed by health-care practitioner

ADRENAL, THYROID, LIVER & DETOX

Boron	Helps remove fluoride	3 mg daily or as directed by health-care practitioner
Brown seaweed (kelp, laminaria) extract	Binds to radioactive particles and escorts them out of the body; also binds to heavy metals and other harmful compounds	4–6 capsules (2 to 3 grams) daily, upon arising
Chlorella	Binds to heavy metals and other toxins	3–9 grams per day 45 minutes before meals
Essiac tea	Potent blend of herbs and bark for detoxification, liver cleansing; kills cancer cells	Prepare as directed by product label
Glutathione Liposomal glutathione	Required for detox; "master antioxidant," injuries, illnesses, stress, toxins, etc.; major factor in overall health and disease resistance	Refer to product label or as directed by health-care practitioner
Homeopathic formulations HVS Laboratories Homeovitics	Liver and detox support	Practitioners only can order
Irish moss	Binds to heavy metals and other toxins and escorts them out of the body	3 capsules 1–2 times daily with 300–350ml of water
MSM	Provides biologically active sulfur, which boosts immune function	3–6 grams daily, divided into 3 doses or as directed by health-care practitioner
Pantethine Vitamin B5	Adrenal support	1,000–2,000 mg daily
Pyrroloquinoline quinone (PQQ)	Mitochondrial support and regeneration, longevity extender, heart and brain protection	20 mg daily or as directed by your health-care practitioner
Ubiquinol Highly bioavailable form of CoQ10	Eliminates free radicals, supports immune system	100–300 mg daily
Zeolites	Helps remove heavy metals, chemicals, radioactive particles, and mold from the body	Take according to instructions on label

CORE SUPPLEMENTS

CLA (conjugated linoleic acid)	Encourages fat burning	1,000 mg 3 times daily
Fish oil	EPA and DHA, long-chain omega-3s; prostaglandins, brain, and nervous system support	1,000–2,000 mg daily after 21-Day Reboot
GLA (gamma linolenic acid) from blackcurrant seed	Stimulates brown fat activity and fat burning, reduces inflammation, optimizes cholesterol, and relieves PMS	360–1,800 mg daily

ADRENAL, THYROID, LIVER & DETOX

Iodine	Optimizes thyroid function	Start with one drop and increase by one drop daily until your basal temperature is at least 36.5°C/97.8°F, or use as directed by your health-care practitioner
Magnesium (full spectrum)	Prevents constipation, supports the heart, enhances sleep, and modulates stress	5 mg per pound of body weight
Multivitamin-multimineral supplement (iron-free or copper-free; iron-free for males)	Overall nutritional support	Take according to instructions on label
Probiotic supplement	Building a healthy microbiome	At least 10 billion CFU; one that includes at least the strains *Lactobacillus plantarum*, *Lactobacillus rhamnosus*, and/or *Lactobacillus gasseri*
Vitamin C	Helps conversion of excess cholesterol into bile; daily C can cut gallstone risk in half	1,000–5,000 mg daily, minimum
Vitamin D	Reduces inflammation, helps heal leaky gut, and positively influences more than 200 genes; cancer prevention	2,000–5,000 IU daily (adjust based on routine blood levels or as directed by health-care practitioner)
Weight-loss support L-carnitine tartrate, choline, chromium	Blood sugar balance, metabolism boost, diminished cravings, increased energy	Take according to instructions on label

MISCELLANEOUS

Bioidentical hormones Estrogen, progesterone, testosterone, DHEA	Hormone balance and prevention of estrogen dominance	As prescribed by health-care practitioner
Black seed oil or powdered black seed	Hashimoto's thyroiditis	2,000 mg or as directed by health-care practitioner
Melatonin	Improves sleep, resets biological clock, cancer protective, antioxidant properties, replenishes levels lowered by exposure to EMFs	1–3 mg before bed or as directed by health-care practitioner

APPENDIX 3: RADICAL READING LIST

MAGAZINES

Gallbladder Newsletter

Produced by Deborah Graefer, creator of GallbladderAttack.com and magna cum laude graduate of Oriental Medicine in San Diego, *Gallbladder Newsletter* has helped thousands all over the world to alleviate symptoms of gallbladder pain. Pertaining to all things related to the gallbladder, it covers such topics as dietary tips, ways to reduce pain or discomfort, removal, what fats to eat, flushes, and more.

www.GallbladderAttack.com

The Health Sciences Institute (HSI) Newsletter

HSI is an independent organization dedicated to uncovering and researching the most urgent advances in modern underground medicine. As a member of the professional advisory panel, I can verify that this cutting-edge newsletter is devoted to presenting extraordinary products to its members before the products hit the marketplace. HSI was the first to break the Ultra H-3 story—the extraordinary product for arthritis, depression, and antiaging. HSI provides private access to hidden cures, powerful discoveries, breakthrough treatments, and advances in modern underground medicine.

http://hsionline.com

First for Women Magazine

With an understanding that women have busy lives, *First for Women* delivers helpful tips and credible information you can't get anywhere else. The magazine provides numerous motivational articles on living a well-rounded life, nurturing family, owning a pet, preparing healthy menus, and just having fun! *First for Women* is very visual, with lots of quick tips and advice that make it easy to read as your schedule allows. I am proud to be a regular contributor.

www.firstforwomen.com

Total Health Online Magazine

The mission of *Total Health Online* magazine is to advocate self-managed natural health, emphasize the importance of becoming the cocaptain of your own health-care team, and address the imperatives to wellness. To achieve this, the magazine provides you, the reader, with the information and resources needed to establish and maintain optimum health as well as to potentiate your immune system in times of crises. I am an associate editor for this outstanding publication.

http://totalhealthmagazine.com

Taste for Life

Taste for Life in-store magazines can be found in health food stores, natural product chains, food co-ops, and supermarkets throughout the US. The publication provides excellent articles on pertinent health issues and serves as an informative educational source on a variety of levels. I am proud to sit on Taste for Life's editorial board. The online website also provides a one-stop natural health resource.

www.tasteforlife.com

Women's World Magazine

A magazine with information and inspiration on topics ranging from food to decor to beauty to nutrition.

http://www.womansworld.com

Nutrition & Healing Newsletter

An author of nine books on topics than range from thyroid disorders to back pain, Dr. Glenn S. Rothfeld has helped thousands of patients find lasting solutions to even the most stubborn health problems. He shares these discoveries monthly in *Dr. Rothfeld's Nutrition & Healing* newsletter.

http://nutritionandhealing.com

BOOKS

Reinventing Your Style: 7 Strategies for Looking Powerful, Dynamic and Inspiring
Jennifer Butler

Discover a reflection of your inner self using a step-by-step guide designed by Jennifer Butler, a master in the art of visual communication. After years of studying great works of art and Mother Nature, Jennifer recognized a natural rhythm, harmony, and symmetry that when applied to human form, brought forth an inner radiance, a natural beauty that cannot be defined by height, weight or ethnic background. These observations are the basis for the seven principles of design presented throughout the title.

Going Against GMOs: The Fast-Growing Movement to Avoid Unnatural Genetically Modified "Foods" to Take Back Our Food

Melissa Diane Smith

Trailblazing nutritionist, Melissa Diane Smith offers a book that is a definitive consumer's guide to understanding genetically modified foods. You'll learn the top 10 reasons to stay away from GMOs; why you have to go against the status quo to avoid GMOs; the Eat GMO-Free Challenge and non-GMO optimal health guidelines; detailed instructions for avoiding GMOs when shopping and eating out; and more than forty-five easy-to-make, non-GMO (and gluten-free) recipes.

The Fungus Link

Doug A. Kaufmann

Learn why so many people have tried and failed to regain their health, simply because they were unaware of the fungus link to their symptoms. This groundbreaking work covers common issues including pain, heart health, allergies, digestive disorders, mental health, women's health, and respiratory challenges.

The End of Acne: How Water Is the Cause of the Modern Acne Epidemic, and the Cure

Melissa Gardner

What if your acne was caused by a toxic waste product that has been added to our American water supply since the 1960s and is in most of our food, especially in processed, packaged, and restaurant foods? Melissa Gardner uncovers fluoride's link to acne as well as conditions, including cysts in your breasts or ovaries, melasma, arthritis, hypothyroidism, thyroid disease, diabetes, PMS, PCOS, tooth decay, osteoporosis, hormonal imbalances or endocrine disruption, heart disease, breast cancer, infertility, and migraines.

The New Fat Flush Plan

Ann Louise Gittleman, PhD, CNS

For over twenty-five years, *Fat Flush* has helped millions of people lose weight, harness the healing powers of foods, reignite metabolism, fight cellulite, and restore the liver and gallbladder while improving their lives. Now, for the first time since its original publication, the acclaimed *New York Times* bestseller has been revised and updated with groundbreaking research, food options, and lifestyle choices to help you achieve lasting weight loss and wellness.

Before the Change

Ann Louise Gittleman, PhD, CNS

Revised and updated, the *New York Times* bestseller is the popular alternative guide for taking charge of your perimenopause, filled with up-to-date research, including the latest information on hormone replacement therapy, mood swings, weight gain, and nutrition for women aged thirty-five and older. The book offers a gentle, proven, incremental program for understanding your body's changes and controlling your symptoms during perimenopause—the period of about ten years leading up to menopause—to help you feel great through this vital phase of life.

Guess What Came to Dinner?

Ann Louise Gittleman, PhD, CNS

Parasites are alive and well in twenty-first-century America. Learn how to protect yourself and your family from this alarming epidemic, which knows no economic or social boundaries. Parasites can masquerade as numerous illnesses, and this book masterfully covers everything you wanted to know and more about the warning signs, the water and food connection, man's best friend, diagnosis, treatment, and prevention.

The Gut Flush Plan

Ann Louise Gittleman, PhD, CNS

The Gut Flush Plan focuses on the new frontier in health care—the new germ warfare—designed to outsmart the hidden invaders and superbugs that are spreading into the community and threatening our health. The book offers concrete steps that protect against the undetected hitchhikers in our food and in our surroundings that take up residence in our gut, making us sick, tired, and bloated. You will learn to fortify your own compromised digestive system against pathogens and parasites, flush out any lingering invaders or toxins, and feed yourself nourishing foods that encourage and rebuild gastrointestinal health.

Super Nutrition for Women

Ann Louise Gittleman, PhD, CNS

Super Nutrition for Women is the perfect book for women in their twenties and thirties who want to learn how to combat PMS, alleviate yeast infections, lose weight, and strengthen their immune system. This book also includes great tips on getting out bad fats, salt, and sugar and boosting the female minerals calcium and iron in your diet. Plus, terrific recipes!

Why Am I Always So Tired?

Ann Louise Gittleman, PhD, CNS

Here is a groundbreaking discovery on the overlooked connection between exhaustion and a copper-zinc imbalance in our body. You will be amazed to read about the copper connection to other disorders, such as hyperactivity, panic attacks, depression, skin conditions, and hormonal imbalances. Copper is found in water pipes, IUDs, and birth control pills (estrogen stockpiles copper) as well as in soy products, chocolate, and regular tea.

Skinny Liver: A Proven Program to Prevent and Reverse the New Silent Epidemic — Fatty Liver Disease

Kristin Kirkpatrick and Ibrahim Hanouneh

Written by two experts in the field and based on the latest research, *Skinny Liver* is an authoritative, easy-to-follow guide that promotes the health of your entire body. Included is a four-week dietary and exercise program, lifestyle changes to get your liver's health back on track, and delicious liver-friendly recipes.

Create a Toxin-Free Body & Home Starting Today

W. Lee Cowden, MD, and Connie Strasheim

You can't escape toxic exposures, but you can reduce their effects . . . starting today. When you eliminate toxins, your mind begins to operate with clarity and sharpness; the aches and pains in your joints and muscles ease; you awaken with new energy, pep and vitality; difficult tasks become easier; you have a new zest and enthusiasm for life; and you sleep more deeply.

Foods That Fit a Unique You

W. Lee Cowden, MD, and Connie Strasheim

In Foods That Fit a Unique You, authors W. Lee Cowden, MD, and Connie Strasheim prove that you can learn how to identify truly healthy foods—and look and feel your best—by taking into account six individual factors, including body pH, food allergies, metabolic type, gastrointestinal function, and your current health condition.

The Wireless Elephant in the Room

Camilla R. G. Rees

Chock-full of research from leading scientific experts, including from Harvard, Columbia, Yale, and other universities, this is a highly informed synopsis of society's new public health predicament. Learn what conditions have been linked to wireless radiation, where you can go for help to measure and minimize exposures, and how to quickly get further up to speed on the basics of safer living in a wireless world.

PEO Solution—Conquering Cancer, Diabetes and Heart Disease with Parent Essential Oils

Brian S. Peskin and Robert Jay Rowen, MD

Learn how practitioners were led astray by the supplement industry, the science of parent essential oils (PEOs) to resolving health issues, and what tools to use to avert potential damage.

The Tapping Solution for Weight Loss & Body Confidence: A Woman's Guide to Stressing Less, Weighing Less, and Loving More

Jessica Ortner

Jessica Ortner is a producer of *The Tapping Solution*, the breakthrough documentary film on EFT/meridian Tapping (www.TheTappingSolution.com). She is the author of *The Tapping Solution for Weight Loss and Body Confidence*—a book based on her revolutionary online program, which has helped more than three thousand women tackle the stress that leads to weight gain.

NOTES

INTRODUCTION: WHY I WROTE THIS BOOK

1. John LaRosa, "Weight Loss Market Sheds Some Dollars in 2013," Marketdarta Enterprises, February 4, 2014, https://www.marketdataenterprises.com/wp-content/uploads/2014/01/Diet-Market-2014-Status-Report.pdf, accessed June 21, 2017.

CHAPTER 1: RESCUING A STALLED METABOLISM

1. "CAS Assigns the 100 Millionth CAS Registry Number to a Substance Designed to Treat Acute Myeloid Leukemia," Chemical Abstracts Service, June 29, 2015, http://www.cas.org/news/media-releases/100-millionth-substance, accessed June 25, 2017.

2. "Heart Disease Facts," Centers for Disease Control and Prevention, August 10, 2015, https://www.cdc.gov/heartdisease/facts.htm, accessed June 22, 2017.

3. E. Fothergill et al., "Persistent Metabolic Adaptation 6 Years After 'The Biggest Loser' Competition," *Obesity* 24 (May 2, 2016): 1612–1619, doi:10.1002/oby.21538, accessed June 23, 2017.

4. "Cell Membranes," October 20, 2012, http://www.biology-pages.info/C/CellMembranes.html, accessed June 22, 2017.

5. Erwin and Hans-Dieter Kuntz, *Hepatology: Textbook and Atlas*, 3rd ed. (Heidelberg: Springer, 2008).

6. Chun-Jung Huang et al., "Obesity-Related Oxidative Stress: The Impact of Physical Activity and Diet Manipulation," *Sports Medicine—Open* 1 (2015): 32, doi:10.1186/s40798-015-0031-y.

7. Surapon Tangvarasittichai, "Oxidative Stress, Insulin Resistance, Dyslipidemia and Type 2 Diabetes Mellitus," *World Journal of Diabetes* 6, no 3 (2015): 456–480, doi:10.4239/wjd.v6.i3.456.

8. Sarah K. Abbott et al., "Fatty Acid Composition of Membrane Bilayers: Importance of Diet Polyunsaturated Fat Balance," *Biochimica et Biophysica Acta (BBA)—Biomembranes* 1818, no. 5 (2012), doi:10.1016/j.bbamem.2012.01.011, accessed June 22, 2017.

9. V. Santilli, A. Bernetti, M. Mangone, and M. Paoloni, "Clinical Definition of Sarcopenia," *Clinical Cases in Mineral and Bone Metabolism* 11, no. 3 (2014): 177–180, doi:10.11138/ccmbm/2014.11.3.177, accessed June 22, 2017.

10. John B. Furness et al., "The Enteric Nervous System and Gastrointestinal Innervation: Integrated Local and Central Control," *Advances in Experimental Medicine and Biology Microbial Endocrinology: The Microbiota-Gut-Brain Axis in Health and Disease* 817 (2014), doi:10.1007/978-1-4939-0897-4_3, accessed June 22, 2017; Adam Hadhazy, "Think Twice: How the Gut's 'Second Brain' Influences Mood and Well-Being," *Scientific American*, February 12, 2010, https://www.scientificamerican.com/article/gut-second-brain/, accessed June 22, 2017.

CHAPTER 2: RADICAL RULE #1: REVAMP YOUR FATS

1. K. L. Stanhope, J.-M. Schwarz, and P. J. Havel, "Adverse Metabolic Effects of Dietary Fructose: Results from Recent Epidemiological, Clinical, and Mechanistic Studies," *Current Opinion in Lipidology* 24, no. 3 (2013): 198–206, doi:10.1097/MOL.0b013e3283613bca; R. H. Lustig, *Fat Chance: Beating the Odds Against Sugar, Processed Food, Obesity, and Disease* (New York: Plume, 2014).

2. B. Best, "Insulin Resistance and Obesity," *Life Extension Magazine*, November 2017, 64–71.

3. "The Official Site of Dr. Pompa," Dr. Pompa, http://drpompa.com, accessed June 22, 2017; "NeuroLipid Research Foundation—Nourish the Membrane, Nourish the Brain," NeuroLipid Research Foundation, http://www.neurolipid.org/, accessed June 22, 2017.

4. J. Bowden and S. T. Sinatra, *The Great Cholesterol Myth: Why Lowering Your Cholesterol Won't Prevent Heart Disease—and the Statin-Free Plan That Will* (Beverly, MA: Fair Winds Press, 2012).

5. B. J. Nicklas et al., "Diet-Induced Weight Loss, Exercise, and Chronic Inflammation in Older, Obese Adults," *American Journal of Clinical Nutrition* 79, no. 4 (April 2004): 544–551, PMID:15051595, http://ajcn.nutrition.org/content/79/4/544.long.

6. "Omega-3 Fatty Acids: An Essential Contribution," *Nutrition Source*, May 26, 2015, https://www.hsph.harvard.edu/nutritionsource/omega-3-fats/, accessed June 22, 2017; "Essential Fatty Acids," Linus Pauling Institute, May 5, 2017, http://lpi.oregonstate.edu/mic/other-nutrients/essential-fatty-acids, accessed June 22, 2017.

7. B. S. Rett and J. Whelan, "Increasing Dietary Linoleic Acid Does Not Increase Tissue Arachidonic Acid Content in Adults Consuming Western-Type Diets: A Systematic Review," *Nutrition & Metabolism* 8 (2011): 36, doi:10.1186/1743-7075-8-36.

8. N. Teicholz, *The Big Fat Surprise: Why Butter, Meat, and Cheese Belong in a Healthy Diet* (New York: Simon & Schuster, 2014).

9. A. M. Hill et al., "Combining Fish Oil Supplements with Regular Aerobic Exercise Improves Body Composition and Cardiovascular Disease Risk Factors," *American Journal of Clinical Nutrition* 85, no. 5 (May 2007): 1267–1274.

10. United Mitochondrial Disease Foundation, https://www.umdf.org/, accessed June 22, 2017.

11. Brian Peskin, "The Perfect Ten—10 Years in 10 Pages: A Decade of Work by Prof. Brian Peskin," http://brianpeskin.com/pdf/about/PeskinPrimer.pdf, accessed June 22, 2017.

12. W. S. Harris et al., "Omega-6 Fatty Acids and Risk for Cardiovascular Disease: A Science Advisory from the American Heart Association Nutrition Subcommittee of the Council on Nutrition, Physical Activity, and Metabolism; Council on Cardiovascular Nursing; and Council on Epidemiology and Prevention," *Circulation* 119, no. 6 (2009), doi:10.1161/circulationaha.108.191627, accessed June 22, 2017.

13. Frank B. Hu et al., "Dietary Fat Intake and the Risk of Coronary Heart Disease in Women," *New England Journal of Medicine* 337, no. 21 (1997), doi:10.1056/nejm199711203372102, accessed June 22, 2017.

14. Stephen D. Anton, Kacey Heekin, Carrah Simkins, and Andres Acosta, "Differential Effects of Adulterated Versus Unadulterated Forms of Linoleic Acid on Cardiovascular Health," *Journal of Integrative Medicine* 11, no. 1 (2013): 2–10, doi:10.3736/jintegrmed2013002, accessed June 22, 2017.

15. I. M. Campbell, D. N. Crozier, and R. B. Caton, "Abnormal Fatty Acid Composition and Impaired Oxygen Supply in Cystic Fibrosis Patients," *Pediatrics* 57, no. 4 (April 1976): 480–486, PMID: 1264543, https://www.ncbi.nlm.nih.gov/pubmed/1264543, accessed June 22, 2017.

16. Ji-Yoon Kim et al., "Growth-Inhibitory and Proapoptotic Effects of Alpha-Linolenic Acid on Estrogen-Positive Breast Cancer Cells," *Annals of the New York Academy of Sciences* 1171, no. 1 (2009), doi:10.1111/j.1749-6632.2009.04897.x, accessed June 22, 2017.

17. A. Cypess et al., "Identification and Importance of Brown Adipose Tissue in Adult Humans," *New England Journal of Medicine* 360, no. 15 (2009): 1509–1517, doi:10.1056/nejmoa0810780, accessed October 29, 2017.

18. U. Risérus, L. Berglund, and B. Vessby, "Conjugated Linoleic Acid (CLA) Reduced Abdominal Adipose Tissue in Obese Middle-Aged Men with Signs of the Metabolic Syndrome: A Randomised Controlled Trial," *International Journal of Obesity* 25, no. 8 (2001): 1129–1135, doi:10.1038/sj.ijo.0801659, accessed June 22, 2017.

19. S. Torabian et al., "Acute Effect of Nut Consumption on Plasma Total Polyphenols, Antioxidant Capacity and Lipid Peroxidation," *Journal of Human Nutrition and Dietetics* 22, no. 1 (2009): 64–71, doi:10.1111/j.1365-277x.2008.00923.x, accessed June 22, 2017; K. N. Aronis et al., "Short-Term Walnut Consumption Increases Circulating Total Adiponectin And Apolipoprotein A Concentrations, but Does Not Affect Markers of Inflammation or Vascular Injury in Obese Humans with the Metabolic Syndrome: Data from a Double-Blinded, Randomized, Placebo-Controlled Study," *Metabolism* 61, no. 4 (2012): 577–582, doi:10.1016/j.metabol.2011.09.008, accessed June 22, 2017; Liya Wu et al., "Walnut-Enriched Diet Reduces Fasting Non-HDL-Cholesterol and Apolipoprotein B in Healthy Caucasian Subjects: A Randomized Controlled Cross-Over Clinical Trial," *Metabolism* 63, no. 3 (2014): 382–391, doi:10.1016/j.metabol.2013.11.005, accessed June 22, 2017.

20. Zhi-Hong Yang, Miyahara Hiroko, and Hatanaka Akimasa, "Chronic Administration of Palmitoleic Acid Reduces Insulin Resistance and Hepatic Lipid Accumulation in KK-Ay Mice with Genetic Type 2 Diabetes," *Lipids in Health and Disease* 10, no. 1 (2011): 120, doi:10.1186/1476-511x-10-120, accessed June 22, 2017.

21. "Omega-7 Protects Against Metabolic Syndrome," LifeExtension.com, April 2014, http://www.lifeextension.com/Magazine/2014/4/Omega-7-Protects-Against-Metabolic-Syndrome/Page-01, accessed June 22, 2017.

22. W. M. A. D. B. Fernando et al., "The Role of Dietary Coconut for the Prevention and Treatment of Alzheimers Disease: Potential Mechanisms of Action," *British Journal of Nutrition* 114, no. 1 (2015): 1–14, doi:10.1017/s0007114515001452, accessed June 22, 2017.

23. V. Van Wymelbeke et al., "Influence of Medium-Chain and Long-Chain Triacylglycerols on the Control of Food Intake in Men," *American Journal of Clinical Nutrition* 68, no. 2 (August 1998): 226–234, https://www.ncbi.nlm.nih.gov/pubmed/9701177, accessed June 22, 2017; Kai Ming Liau, Yeong Yeh Lee, Chen Chee Keong, and G. Rasool Aida Hanum, "An Open-Label Pilot Study to Assess the Efficacy and Safety of Virgin Coconut Oil in Reducing Visceral Adiposity," *ISRN Pharmacology* 2011 (2011): 1–7, doi:10.5402/2011/949686, accessed June 22, 2017; M. L. Assunção, H. S. Ferreira, A. F. dos Santos, et al., "Effects of Dietary Coconut Oil on the Biochemical and Anthropometric Profiles of Women Presenting Abdominal Obesity," *Lipids* 44 (2009): 593, doi:10.1007/s11745-009-3306-6, accessed June 20, 2017.

24. J. A. Paniagua et al., "Monounsaturated Fat-Rich Diet Prevents Central Body Fat Distribution and Decreases Postprandial Adiponectin Expression Induced by a Carbohydrate-Rich Diet in Insulin-Resistant Subjects," *Diabetes Care* 30, no. 7 (2007): 1717–1723, doi:10.2337/dc06-2220, accessed October 29, 2017.

25. Maddie Oatman, "Your Olive Oil Could Be Fake," *Mother Jones*, January 19, 2017, http://www.motherjones.com/environment/2016/08/olive-oil-fake-larry-olmsted-food-fraud-usda/, accessed June 22, 2017; "Olive Oil Fraud Articles and Updates," *Olive Oil Times*, https://www.oliveoiltimes.com/tag/olive-oil-fraud?page=3, accessed June 22, 2017.

26. C. A. Daley et al., "A Review of Fatty Acid Profiles and Antioxidant Content in Grass-Fed and Grain-Fed Beef," *Nutrition Journal* 9 (2010): 10, doi:10.1186/1475-2891-9-10.

27. Edward Kane, "4:1 Oil—the Right Stuff," *BodyBio Bulletin*, 2008, http://blog.bodybio.com/download/why-41-ratio-oil/?wpdmdl=1268, accessed June 22, 2017.

CHAPTER 3: RADICAL RULE #2: RESTORE YOUR GALLBLADDER

1. C. M. St. George, J. C. Russell, and E. A. Shaffer, "Effects of Obesity on Bile Formation and Biliary Lipid Secretion in the Genetically Obese JCR:LA-Corpulent Rat," *Hepatology* 20 (1994): 1541–1547, doi:10.1002/hep.1840200625, accessed June 23, 2017.

2. Yan Zheng et al., "Gallstones and Risk of Coronary Heart Disease," *Arteriosclerosis, Thrombosis, and Vascular Biology* (2016), originally published August 18, 2016, https://doi.org/10.1161/ATVBAHA.116.307507, accessed June 23, 2017.

3. G. E. Njeze, "Gallstones," *Nigerian Journal of Surgery: Official Publication of the Nigerian Surgical Research Society* 19, no. 2 (2013): 49–55, doi:10.4103/1117-6806.119236, accessed June 23, 2017.

4. J. R. Thornton, P. M. Emmett, and K. W. Heaton, "Diet and Gall Stones: Effects of Refined and Unrefined Carbohydrate Diets on Bile Cholesterol Saturation and Bile Acid Metabolism," *Gut* 24, no. 1 (1983): 2–6, doi:10.1136/gut.24.1.2, accessed June 23, 2017; L. M. Stinton and E. A. Shaffer, "Epidemiology of Gallbladder Disease: Cholelithiasis and Cancer," *Gut and Liver* 6, no. 2 (2012): 172–187, doi:10.5009/gnl.2012.6.2.172, accessed June 23, 2017.

5. A. A. Siddiqui et al., "A Previous Cholecystectomy Increases the Risk of Developing Advanced Adenomas of the Colon," *Southern Medical Journal* 102, no. 11 (2009): 1111–1115, http://www.medscape.com/viewarticle/712494_4, accessed June 23, 2017; Charles Thomas, Johan Auwerx, and Kristina Schoonjans, "Bile Acids and the Membrane Bile Acid Receptor TGR5—Connecting Nutrition and Metabolism," *Thyroid* 18, no. 2 (February 2008): 167–174, https://doi.org/10.1089/thy.2007.0255, accessed June 23, 2017.

6. M.-S. Kwak et al., "Cholecystectomy Is Independently Associated with Nonalcoholic Fatty Liver Disease in an Asian Population," *World Journal of Gastroenterology* 21, no. 20 (2015): 6287–6295, doi:10.3748/wjg.v21.i20.6287, accessed June 23, 2017; Chao Shen, "Association of Cholecystectomy with Metabolic Syndrome in a Chinese Population," *PLoS ONE* 9, no. 2 (2014), doi:10.1371/journal.pone.0088189, accessed June 23, 2017.

7. J. R. F. Walters and S. S. Pattni, "Managing Bile Acid Diarrhea," *Therapeutic Advances in Gastroenterology* 3, no. 6 (2010): 349–357, doi:10.1177/1756283X10377126, accessed June 23, 2017.

8. H. Ma and M. E. Patti, "Bile Acids, Obesity, and the Metabolic Syndrome" *Best Practice & Research Clinical Gastroenterology* 28, no. 4 (2014): 573–583, doi:10.1016/j.bpg.2014.07.004, accessed June 23, 2017.

9. "Choline," Linus Pauling Institute, January 3, 2017, http://lpi.oregonstate.edu/mic/other-nutrients/choline#cardiovascular-disease-prevention, accessed June 23, 2017.

10. A. L. Guerrerio, "Choline Intake in a Large Cohort of Patients with Nonalcoholic Fatty Liver Disease," *American Journal of Clinical Nutrition* 95, no. 4 (2012): 892–900, doi:10.3945/ajcn.111.020156, accessed June 23, 2017.

11. A. M. Mourad et al., "Influence of Soy Lecithin Administration on Hypercholesterolemia," *Cholesterol* (2010): 824813, doi:10.1155/2010/824813, accessed June 23, 2017; T. A. Wilson, C. M. Meservey, and R. J. Nicolosi, "Soy Lecithin Reduces Plasma Lipoprotein Cholesterol and Early Atherogenesis in Hypercholesterolemic Monkeys and Hamsters: Beyond Linoleate," *Atherosclerosis* 140, no. 1 (September 1998): 147–153, doi:http://dx.doi.org/10.1016/S0021-9150(98)00132-4, accessed June 23, 2017; D. Küllenberg et al. "Health Effects of Dietary Phospholipids," *Lipids in Health and Disease* 11 (2012): 3, doi:10.1186/1476-511X-11-3, accessed June 23, 2017; Marie-Josée Leblanc, "The Role of Dietary Choline in the Beneficial Effects of Lecithin on the Secretion of Biliary Lipids in Rats," *Biochimica et Biophysica Acta (BBA)—Lipids and Lipid Metabolism* 1393, no. 2–3 (1998): 223–234, doi:10.1016/s0005-2760(98)00072-1, accessed June 23, 2017.

12. W. H. W. Tang et al., "Intestinal Microbial Metabolism of Phosphatidylcholine and Cardiovascular Risk," *New England Journal of Medicine* 368, no. 17 (2013): 1575–1584, doi:10.1056/nejmoa1109400, accessed June 23, 2017.

13. "Epidemiology of the IBD," Centers for Disease Control and Prevention, March 31, 2015, https://www.cdc.gov/ibd/ibd-epidemiology.htm, accessed June 23, 2017.

14. A. C. Dukowicz, B. E. Lacy, and G. M. Levine, "Small Intestinal Bacterial Overgrowth: A Comprehensive Review," *Gastroenterology & Hepatology* 3, no. 2 (2007): 112–122, PMCID: PMC3099351, accessed June 23, 2017.

15. M. F. Leitzmann et al., "Recreational Physical Activity and the Risk of Cholecystectomy in Women," *New England Journal of Medicine* 342, no. 3 (2000): 212–214, doi:10.1056/nejm200001203420313, accessed June 23, 2017.

16. Dr. Terry Wahls (July 13, 2015), Ann Louise Gittleman, PhD, CNS (June 6, 2017), and Alice Abler (November 3, 2016), "Debunking the Myths About GERD," Price Pottenger, May 23, 2017, https://price-pottenger.org/journals/debunking-myths-about-gerd, accessed June 23, 2017.

17. J. A. Simon and E. S. Hudes, "Serum Ascorbic Acid and Gallbladder Disease Prevalence Among US Adults," *Archives of Internal Medicine* 160, no. 7 (2000): 931, doi:10.1001/archinte.160.7.931, accessed June 23, 2017; E. Ginter, "Cholesterol: Vitamin C Controls Its Transformation to Bile Acids," *Science* 179, no. 4074 (1973): 702–704, doi:10.1126/science.179.4074.702, accessed June 23, 2017.

18. Jonathan Wright, *Why Stomach Acid Is Good for You: Natural Relief from Heartburn, Indigestion, Reflux and GERD* (Lanham, MD: M. Evans & Co., 2001).

19. "General Information/Press Room," American Thyroid Association, http://www.thyroid.org/media-main/about-hypothyroidism/, accessed June 23, 2017.

20. J. Laukkarinen, J. Sand, and I. Nordback, "The Underlying Mechanisms: How Hypothyroidism Affects the Formation of Common Bile Duct Stones—A Review," *HPB Surgery* 2012 (January 2012): 1–7, doi:10.1155/2012/102825, accessed June 23, 2017.

21. J. Laukkarinen et al., "Increased Prevalence of Subclinical Hypothyroidism in Common Bile Duct Stone Patients," *Journal of Clinical Endocrinology & Metabolism* 92, no. 11 (2007): 4260–4264, doi: 10.1210/jc.2007-1316, accessed June 23, 2017.

22. Mitsuhiro Watanabe, "Bile Acids Induce Energy Expenditure by Promoting Intracellular Thyroid Hormone Activation," *Nature* 439, no. 7075 (2006): 484–489, doi:10.1038/nature04330, accessed June 23, 2017; Johann Ockenga et al., "Plasma Bile Acids Are Associated with Energy Expenditure and Thyroid Function in Humans," *Journal of Clinical Endocrinology & Metabolism* 97, no. 2 (2012): 535–542, doi: 10.1210/jc.2011-2329, accessed June 23, 2017; Thomas, Auwerx, and Schoonjans, "Bile Acids and the Membrane Bile Acid Receptor TGR5."

23. Craig Gustafson and Antonio C. Bianco, MD, PhD, "Is T4 Enough for Patients with Hypothyroid Dysfunction? *Integrative Medicine: A Clinician's Journal* 13, no. 3 (2014): 20–22, accessed June 23, 2017; A. C. Bianco, "Cracking the Code for Thyroid Hormone Signaling," *Transactions of the American Clinical and Climatological Association* 124 (2013): 26–35, PMCID: PMC3715916, accessed June 23, 2017.

24. Johanna Laukkarinen, "Is Bile Flow Reduced in Patients with Hypothyroidism?," *Surgery* 133, no. 3 (2003): 288–293, doi:10.1067/msy.2003.77, accessed June 23, 2017.

25. J. Laukkarinen, "Mechanism of the Prorelaxing Effect of Thyroxine on the Sphincter of Oddi," *Scandinavian Journal of Gastroenterology* 37, no. 6 (2002): 667–673, doi:10.1080/00365520212492, accessed June 23, 2017.

26. "Autoimmune Disease: Stop Your Body's Self-Attack," *Dr. Mark Hyman*, April 20, 2010, http://drhyman.com/blog/2010/04/20/autoimmune-disease-stop-your-body-from-attacking-itself/, accessed June 23, 2017.

27. Roxanne Nelson, "Autoimmune Diseases Among Top Killers of Younger Women," WebMD, September 1, 2000, http://www.webmd.com/women/news/20000901/autoimmune-diseases-among-top-killers-of-younger-women#1, accessed June 23, 2017.

28. Dana Trentini, "90% of People Taking Thyroid Hormones Will Fail to Feel Normal: Why?" *Hypothyroid Mom*, http://hypothyroidmom.com/90-of-people-taking-thyroid-hormones-will-fail-to-feel-normal-why/, accessed June 23, 2017.

29. T. Akamizu and N. Amino, "Hashimoto's Thyroiditis" (updated July 17, 2017), in *Endotext*, ed. L. J. De Groot, G. Chrousos, K. Dungan, et al. (South Dartmouth, MA: MDText.com, Inc., 2000), available from https://www.ncbi.nlm.nih.gov/books/NBK285557/.

30. T. Akamizu, N. Amino, and L. J. DeGroot, "Hashimoto's Thyroiditis" (updated December 20, 2013), in *Endotext*, ed. DeGroot, Chrousos, Dungan, et al., accessed June 23, 2017; K. Zaletel and S. Gaberšček, "Hashimoto's Thyroiditis: From Genes to the Disease," *Current Genomics* 12, no. 8 (2011): 576–588, doi:10.2174/138920211798120763, accessed June 23, 2017.

31. R. Valentino et al., "Markers of Potential Coeliac Disease in Patients with Hashimoto's Thyroiditis," *European Journal of Endocrinology* 146, no. 4 (April 2002): 479–483, PMID:11916614, http://www.eje-online.org/content/146/4/479.long, accessed June 23, 2017.

32. M. A. Farhangi et al., "The Effects of Nigella Sativa on Thyroid Function, Serum Vascular Endothelial Growth Factor (VEGF)-1, Nesfatin-1 and Anthropometric Features in Patients with Hashimoto's Thyroiditis: A Randomized Controlled Trial," *BMC Complementary and Alternative Medicine* 16 (2016): 471, doi:10.1186/s12906-016-1432-2, accessed June 23, 2017.

33. "Allergic Reaction—Gallbladder Problems," Allergy Self Help, http://allergy-book.blogspot.com/2007/11/allergic-reaction-gallbladder-problems.html, accessed June 25, 2017.

34. "Gallstones," *New York Times*, August 26, 2013, http://www.nytimes.com/health /guides/disease/gallstones/risk-factors.html, accessed June 23, 2017.

35. J. J. DiNicolantonio and S. C. Lucan, "The Wrong White Crystals: Not Salt but Sugar as Aetiological in Hypertension and Cardiometabolic Disease," *Open Heart* 1, no, 1 (2014): e000167, doi:10.1136/openhrt-2014-000167, accessed June 23, 2017.

36. "Dandy Tummy Bitters Recipe," Mountain Rose Herbs, https://blog.mountainrose herbs.com/dandy-tummy-bitters-recipe, accessed June 23, 2017.

37. "Do Angostura Bitters Contain Angostura?" CulinaryLore.com, February 4, 2015, http://www.culinarylore.com/drinks:do-angostura-bitters-contain-angostura, accessed June 23, 2017.

38. Nobuyo Tsuboyama-Kasaoka et al., "Taurine (2-Aminoethanesulfonic Acid) Deficiency Creates a Vicious Circle Promoting Obesity," *Endocrinology* 147, no. 7 (2006): 3276–3284, doi: 10.1210/en.2005-1007, accessed June 23, 2017.

39. Leigh Erin Connealy, *The Cancer Revolution: A Groundbreaking Program to Reverse and Prevent Cancer* (Boston, MA: Da Capo Lifelong, 2017).

40. T. Walcher et al., "Vitamin C Supplement Use May Protect Against Gallstones: An Observational Study on a Randomly Selected Population," *BMC Gastroenterology* 9 (2009): 74, doi:10.1186/1471-230X-9-74, accessed June 23, 2017.

41. L. K. Helbronn et al., "Alternate-Day Fasting in Nonobese Subjects: Effects on Body Weight, Body Composition, and Energy Metabolism," *American Journal of Clinical Nutrition* 81, no. 1 (January 2005): 69–73, https://www.ncbi.nlm.nih.gov/pubmed/15640462, accessed June 23, 2017; Adrianne R. Barnosky, "Intermittent Fasting vs Daily Calorie Restriction for Type 2 Diabetes Prevention: A Review of Human Findings," *Translational Research* 164, no. 4 (2014): 302–311, doi:10.1016/j.trsl.2014.05.013, accessed June 23, 2017.

42. M. Alirezaei, "Short-Term Fasting Induces Profound Neuronal Autophagy," *Autophagy* 6, no. 6 (2010): 702–710, doi:10.4161/auto.6.6.12376, accessed June 23, 2017.

43. Hallie Levine, "Your Metabolism: A User's Manual," *Health*, November 2016, 109–112.

44. Kris Gunnars, "Intermittent Fasting 101—The Ultimate Beginner's Guide," *Authority Nutrition*, June 4, 2017, https://authoritynutrition.com/intermittent-fasting-guide/, accessed June 23, 2017.

CHAPTER 4: RADICAL RULE #3: REBUILD YOUR MUSCLES

1. "Appendix 7. Nutritional Goals for Age-Sex Groups Based on Dietary Reference Intakes and Dietary Guidelines Recommendations," Nutritional Goals for Age-Sex Groups Based on Dietary Reference Intakes and Dietary Guidelines Recommendations—2015–2020 Dietary Guidelines, https://health.gov/dietaryguidelines/2015/guidelines/appendix-7/, accessed June 24, 2017.

2. Christopher A. Taylor et al., "Traumatic Brain Injury–Related Emergency Department Visits, Hospitalizations, and Deaths—United States, 2007 and 2013," *MMWR Surveillance Summaries* 66, SS-9 (2017): 1–16, doi: http://dx.doi.org/10.15585/mmwr.ss6609a1.

3. L. Wandrag et al., "Impact of Supplementation with Amino Acids or Their Metabolites on Muscle Wasting in Patients with Critical Illness or Other Muscle Wasting Illness: A Systematic Review," *Journal of Human Nutrition and Dietetics* 28, no. 4 (2014): 313–330, doi:10.1111

/jhn.12238, accessed June 24, 2017; G. Marchesini et al., "Branched-Chain Amino Acid Supplementation in Patients with Liver Diseases," *Journal of Nutrition* 135, no. 6 Suppl. (June 2005): 1596S–1601S, http://jn.nutrition.org/content/135/6/1596S.long, accessed June 24, 2017.

4. Geoffrey M. Cooper, *The Cell: A Molecular Approach*, 2nd ed. (Sunderland, MA: Sinauer Associates; 2000), available from https://www.ncbi.nlm.nih.gov/books/NBK9928/, accessed June 24, 2017; "Cell Biology@Yale," Medcell.med.yale.edu, http://medcell.med.yale.edu/lectures/introduction_cell_membrane.php, accessed June 24, 2017.

5. G. A. Garden and A. R. La Spada, "Intercellular (Mis)communication in Neurodegenerative Disease," *Neuron* 73, no. 5 (2012): 886–901, doi:10.1016/j.neuron.2012.02.017, accessed June 24, 2017.

6. I.-S. Cheng et al., "The Supplementation of Branched-Chain Amino Acids, Arginine, and Citrulline Improves Endurance Exercise Performance in Two Consecutive Days," *Journal of Sports Science & Medicine* 15, no. 3 (2016): 509–515, https://www.ncbi.nlm.nih.gov/pmc/articles/PMC4974864/, accessed June 24, 2017.

7. E. Blomstrand, "Branched-Chain Amino Acids Activate Key Enzymes in Protein Synthesis After Physical Exercise," *Journal of Nutrition* 136, no. 1 Suppl. (January 2006): 269S–273S, https://www.ncbi.nlm.nih.gov/pubmed/16365096, accessed June 24, 2017.

8. L.-Q. Qin et al., "Higher Branched-Chain Amino Acid Intake Is Associated with a Lower Prevalence of Being Overweight or Obese in Middle-Aged East Asian and Western Adults," *Journal of Nutrition* 141, no. 2 (2011): 249–254, doi:10.3945/jn.110.128520, accessed June 24, 2017.

9. G. Howatson et al., "Exercise-Induced Muscle Damage Is Reduced in Resistance-Trained Males by Branched Chain Amino Acids: A Randomized, Double-Blind, Placebo Controlled Study," *Journal of the International Society of Sports Nutrition* 9 (2012): 20, doi:10.1186/1550-2783-9-20, accessed June 24, 2017.

10. Shinobu Nishitani et al., "Branched-Chain Amino Acids Improve Glucose Metabolism in Rats with Liver Cirrhosis," *American Journal of Physiology—Gastrointestinal and Liver Physiology* 288, no. 6 (June 2005): G1292–G1300, doi:10.1152/ajpgi.00510.2003, accessed June 24, 2017.

11. J. J. Hulmi, C. M. Lockwood, and J. R. Stout, "Effect of Protein/Essential Amino Acids and Resistance Training on Skeletal Muscle Hypertrophy: A Case for Whey Protein," *Nutrition & Metabolism* 7 (2010): 51, doi:10.1186/1743-7075-7-51, accessed June 24, 2017.

12. David Williams, MD, "The Health Benefits of Whey | Dr. Williams," Digestion & Joint Health Tips & Vitamin Products, https://www.drdavidwilliams.com/the-health-benefits-of-whey, accessed June 24, 2017.

13. C. B. Newgard, "Interplay Between Lipids and Branched-Chain Amino Acids in Development of Insulin Resistance," *Cell Metabolism* 15, no. 5 (2012): 606–614, doi:10.1016/j.cmet.2012.01.024, accessed June 24, 2017.

14. L. Wandrag et al., "Impact of Supplementation with Amino Acids or Their Metabolites on Muscle Wasting in Patients with Critical Illness or Other Muscle Wasting Illness: A Systematic Review," *Journal of Human Nutrition and Dietetics* 28 (2015): 313–330, doi:10.1111/jhn.12238, accessed June 24, 2017.

15. H. Zhou and S. Huang, "Role of mTOR Signaling in Tumor Cell Motility, Invasion and Metastasis," *Current Protein & Peptide Science* 12, no. 1 (2011): 30–42, PMCID:

PMC3410744, https://www.ncbi.nlm.nih.gov/pmc/articles/PMC3410744/, accessed June 24, 2017.

16. A. C. Knapp et al., "Effect of Carnitine Deprivation on Carnitine Homeostasis and Energy Metabolism in Mice with Systemic Carnitine Deficiency," *Annals of Nutrition and Metabolism* 52 (2008): 136–144, doi:10.1159/000127390, accessed January 16, 2018.

17. A. Biswas, P. I. Oh, G. E. Faulkner, R. R. Bajaj, M. A. Silver, M. S. Mitchell et al., "Sedentary Time and Its Association with Risk for Disease Incidence, Mortality, and Hospitalization in Adults: A Systematic Review and Meta-Analysis," *Annals of Internal Medicine* 162 (2015): 123–132, doi: 10.7326/M14-1651.

CHAPTER 5: RADICAL RULE #4: REPAIR YOUR GUT

1. J. Lloyd-Price, G. Abu-Ali, and C. Huttenhower, "The Healthy Human Microbiome," *Genome Medicine* 8 (2016): 51, doi:10.1186/s13073-016-0307-y, accessed June 24, 2017; S. Qi, M. Chang, and L. Chai, "The Fungal Mycobiome and Its Interaction with Gut Bacteria in the Host," *International Journal of Molecular Sciences* 18, no. 2 (2017): 330, doi:10.3390/ijms18020330, accessed June 25, 2017; E. Delwart, "The Human Virome," *The Scientist Magazine*, November 1, 2016, http://www.the-scientist.com/?articles.view/articleNo/47291/title/Viruses-of-the-Human-Body/, accessed June 24, 2017.

2. R. Sender, S. Fuchs, and R. Milo, "Revised Estimates for the Number of Human and Bacteria Cells in the Body," bioRxiv 036103; doi: https://doi.org/10.1101/036103, now published in *PLOS Biology*, doi: 10.1371/journal.pbio.1002533, accessed June 24, 2017.

3. R. Eveleth, "There Are 37.2 Trillion Cells in Your Body," *Smithsonian Magazine*, October 24, 2013, http://www.smithsonianmag.com/smart-news/there-are-372-trillion-cells-in-your-body-4941473/, accessed June 24, 2017.

4. F. Karlsson et al., "Assessing the Human Gut Microbiota in Metabolic Diseases," *Diabetes* 62, no. 10 (2013): 3341–3349, doi:10.2337/db13-0844, accessed January 30, 2018; C. M. Ferreira et al., "The Central Role of the Gut Microbiota in Chronic Inflammatory Diseases," *Journal of Immunology Research* 2014 (2014);689492, doi:10.1155/2014/689492, accessed January 30, 2018.

5. F. D. Karlsson et al., "Symptomatic Atherosclerosis Is Associated with an Altered Gut Metagenome," *Nature Communications* 3 (2012): 1245, doi:10.1038/ncomms2266, accessed June 25, 2017.

6. M. C. Dao et al., "*Akkermansia muciniphila* and Improved Metabolic Health During a Dietary Intervention in Obesity: Relationship with Gut Microbiome Richness and Ecology," *Gut* 65 (2016): 426–436, accessed October 30, 2017.

7. L. Guo et al., "PGRP-SC2 Promotes Gut Immune Homeostasis to Limit Commensal Dysbiosis and Extend Lifespan," *Cell* 156, no. 1–2 (January 16, 2014): 109–122, doi: http://dx.doi.org/10.1016/j.cell.2013.12.018, accessed June 24, 2017.

8. M. Sanchez et al., "Effect of Lactobacillus rhamnosus CGMCC1.3724 Supplementation on Weight Loss and Maintenance in Obese Men and Women," *British Journal of Nutrition* 111, no. 8 (2013): 1507–1519, doi:10.1017/s0007114513003875, accessed June 24, 2017.

9. S.-P. Jung et al., "Effect of *Lactobacillus gasseri* BNR17 on Overweight and Obese Adults: A Randomized, Double-Blind Clinical Trial," *Korean Journal of Family Medicine* 34, no. 2 (2013): 80–89, doi:10.4082/kjfm.2013.34.2.80, accessed June 25, 2017.

10. M. Mar Rodríguez et al., "Obesity Changes the Human Gut Mycobiome," *Nature News* (October 12, 2015), http://www.nature.com/articles/srep14600, accessed January 30, 2018; M. Ghannoum, "The Mycobiome," *The Scientist* (February 1, 2016) http://www.the-scientist.com/?articles.view/articleNo/45153/title/The-Mycobiome/, accessed January 30, 2018.

11. S. O. Fetissov, "Role of the Gut Microbiota in Host Appetite Control: Bacterial Growth to Animal Feeding Behavior," *Nature Reviews Endocrinology* 13, no. 1 (2016): 11–25, doi:10.1038/nrendo.2016.150, accessed October 16, 2017.

12. Kelly Brogan, MD, "Psychobiotics: Bacteria for Your Brain?" GreenMedInfo (blog entry), July 2, 2015, http://www.greenmedinfo.com/blog/psychobiotics-bacteria-your-brain, accessed June 25, 2017.

13. "Facts and Statistics," FARE, https://www.foodallergy.org/facts-and-stats, accessed June 25, 2017.

14. "Intestinal Bacteria Influence Food Allergies," *ScienceDaily*, September 7, 2016, https://www.sciencedaily.com/releases/2016/09/160907125125.htm, accessed June 25, 2017.

15. J. Hollon et al., "Effect of Gliadin on Permeability of Intestinal Biopsy Explants from Celiac Disease Patients and Patients with Non-Celiac Gluten Sensitivity," *Nutrients* 7, no. 3 (2015): 1565–1576, doi:10.3390/nu7031565, accessed June 25, 2017.

16. H. J. Freeman, "Hepatobiliary And Pancreatic Disorders in Celiac Disease," *World Journal of Gastroenterology* 12, no. 10 (2006): 1503, doi:10.3748/wjg.v12.i10.1503, accessed June 25, 2017.

17. S. R. Gundry, *The Plant Paradox: The Hidden Dangers in "Healthy" Foods That Cause Disease and Weight Gain* (New York: Harper Wave, 2017).

18. "Genetically Engineered Foods May Cause Rising Food Allergies," Organic Consumers Association, May 1, 2007, https://www.organicconsumers.org/news/genetically-engineered-foods-may-cause-rising-food-allergies, accessed June 25, 2017.

19. M. B. Abou-Donia et al., "Splenda Alters Gut Microflora and Increases Intestinal P-Glycoprotein and Cytochrome P-450 in Male Rats," *Journal of Toxicology and Environmental Health, Part A* 71, no. 21 (2008): 1415–1429, doi:10.1080/15287390802328630, accessed June 25, 2017.

20. V. Leone et al., "Effects of Diurnal Variation of Gut Microbes and High Fat Feeding on Host Circadian Clock Function and Metabolism," *Cell Host & Microbe* 17, no. 5 (2015): 681–689, doi:10.1016/j.chom.2015.03.006, accessed June 25, 2017.

21. B. J. Hardick, "Is Xylitol a Friend or Foe?" DrHardick.com, April 14, 2017, http://drhardick.com/xylitol-sugar-alcohols, accessed June 25, 2017.

22. M. Kumar et al., "Cholesterol-Lowering Probiotics as Potential Biotherapeutics for Metabolic Diseases," *Experimental Diabetes Research* 2012 (2012): 902917, doi:10.1155/2012/902917, accessed June 25, 2017.

23. A. T. Stefka et al., "Commensal Bacteria Protect Against Food Allergen Sensitization," *Proceedings of the National Academy of Sciences of the United States of America* 111, no. 36 (2014): 13145–13150, doi:10.1073/pnas.1412008111, accessed June 25, 2017.

24. J. Tan et al., "Dietary Fiber and Bacterial SCFA Enhance Oral Tolerance and Protect Against Food Allergy Through Diverse Cellular Pathways," *Cell Reports* 15, no. 12 (2016): 2809–2824, doi:10.1016/j.celrep.2016.05.047, accessed June 25, 2017.

25. A. Trompette et al., "Gut Microbiota Metabolism of Dietary Fiber Influences Allergic Airway Disease and Hematopoiesis," *Nature Medicine* 20, no. 2 (2014): 159–166, doi:10.1038/nm.3444, accessed June 25, 2017.

26. T. Raftery et al., "Effects of Vitamin D Supplementation on Intestinal Permeability, Cathelicidin and Disease Markers in Crohn's Disease: Results from a Randomised Double-Blind Placebo-Controlled Study," *United European Gastroenterology Journal* 3, no. 3 (2015): 294–302, doi:10.1177/2050640615572176, accessed June 25, 2017; S. Chen et al., "1,25-Di-hydroxyvitamin D3 Preserves Intestinal Epithelial Barrier Function from TNF-α Induced Injury via Suppression of NF-kB p65 Mediated MLCK-P-MLC Signaling Pathway," *Biochemical and Biophysical Research Communications* 460, no. 3 (2015): 873–878, doi:10.1016/j.bbrc.2015.03.125, accessed June 25, 2017.

27. C. Staley et al., "Successful Resolution of Recurrent Clostridium Difficile Infection Using Freeze-Dried, Encapsulated Fecal Microbiota; Pragmatic Cohort Study," *American Journal of Gastroenterology* 112, no. 6 (2017): 940–947, doi:10.1038/ajg.2017.6, accessed June 25, 2017.

28. A. Vrieze et al., "Transfer of Intestinal Microbiota from Lean Donors Increases Insulin Sensitivity in Individuals with Metabolic Syndrome," *Gastroenterology* 143, no. 4 (2012), doi:10.1053/j.gastro.2012.06.031, accessed June 25, 2017.

29. The Power of Poop, http://thepowerofpoop.com/, accessed June 25, 2017.

CHAPTER 6: RADICAL RULE #5: REDUCE YOUR TOXIC LOAD

1. R. E. Brown et al., "Secular Differences in the Association Between Caloric Intake, Macronutrient Intake, and Physical Activity with Obesity," *Obesity Research & Clinical Practice* 10, no. 3 (2016): 243–255, doi:10.1016/j.orcp.2015.08.007, accessed June 25, 2017.

2. "Body Burden: The Pollution in Newborns," Environmental Working Group, July 14, 2005, http://www.ewg.org/research/body-burden-pollution-newborns, accessed June 25.

3. B. C. Wilding, K. Curtis, K. and Welker-Hood, "Hazardous Chemicals in Health Care," Physicians for Social Responsibility, http://www.psr.org/assets/pdfs/hazardous-chemicals-in-health-care.pdf, accessed June 25, 2017.

4. "Drugs in the Water," Harvard Health, Accessed October 17, 2017. https://www.health.harvard.edu/newsletter_article/drugs-in-the-water.

5. S. Özen and S. Darcan, "Effects of Environmental Endocrine Disruptors on Pubertal Development," *Journal of Clinical Research in Pediatric Endocrinology* 3, no. 1 (2011): 1–6, doi:10.4274/jcrpe.v3i1.01, accessed June 26, 2017.

6. "Dirty Dozen Endocrine Disruptors," Environmental Working Group, http://www.ewg.org/research/dirty-dozen-list-endocrine-disruptors, accessed June 26, 2017.

7. "Health Effects," Fluoride Action Network, http://fluoridealert.org/issues/health/, accessed June 26, 2017.

8. "Pesticides," Fluoride Action Network, http://fluoridealert.org/researchers/pesticide/, accessed June 26, 2017.

9. E. Malinowska et al., "Assessment of Fluoride Concentration and Daily Intake by Human from Tea and Herbal Infusions," *Food and Chemical Toxicology* 46, no. 3 (2008): 1055–1061, doi:10.1016/j.fct.2007.10.039, accessed June 26, 2017.

10. "The Japanese Secret That Doubles Fat Loss," *First for Women Magazine*, November 13, 2017, 26–27.

11. Gadolinium Toxicity, https://gadoliniumtoxicity.com, accessed October 27, 2017.

12. C. Exley, "Aluminum Should Now Be Considered a Primary Etiological Factor in Alzheimer's Disease," *Journal of Alzheimer's Disease Reports* 1, no. 1 (June 8, 2017): 23–25, doi:10.3233/ADR-170010, accessed June 26, 2017.

13. "Nickel—Toxicity and Detoxing," DoctorMyhill, http://www.drmyhill.co.uk/wiki /Nickel_-_toxicity_and_detoxing, accessed June 26, 2017.

14. Y.-H. Chiou et al., "Nickel Accumulation in Lung Tissues Is Associated with Increased Risk of p53 Mutation in Lung Cancer Patients," *Environmental and Molecular Mutagenesis* 55 ((2014): 624–632, doi:10.1002/em.21867, accessed June 26, 2017.

15. S. Olson, "E-Cigs' Dangerous Duo: The Lowdown on Nickel and Chromium," *Medical Daily*, September 2, 2014, http://www.medicaldaily.com/e-cigarettes-emit-levels-nickel -and-chromium-4-times-higher-tobacco-smoke-300704, accessed June 26, 2017.

16. L. Yin et al., "Associations of Blood Mercury, Inorganic Mercury, Methyl Mercury and Bisphenol A with Dental Surface Restorations in the U.S. Population, NHANES 2003–2004 and 2010–2012," *Ecotoxicology and Environmental Safety* 134 (2016): 213–225, doi:10.1016/j.ecoenv.2016.09.001, accessed June 26, 2017.

17. J. T. Salonen et al., "Intake of Mercury from Fish, Lipid Peroxidation, and the Risk of Myocardial Infarction and Coronary, Cardiovascular, and Any Death in Eastern Finnish Men," *Circulation* 91, no. 3 (1995): 645–655, doi:10.1161/01.cir.91.3.645, accessed June 26, 2017.

18. "Health Effects of Lead Exposure," Oregon Department of Human Services, http:// www.oregon.gov/oha/ph/HealthyEnvironments/HealthyNeighborhoods/LeadPoisoning /MedicalProvidersLaboratories/Documents/introhealtheffectsmedicalprovider.pdf, accessed June 26, 2017.

19. N. D. Vaziri, "Mechanisms of Lead-Induced Hypertension and Cardiovascular Disease," *American Journal of Physiology—Heart and Circulatory Physiology* 295, no. 2 (August 2008): H454–H465, doi:10.1152/ajpheart.00158.2008, accessed January 17, 2018.

20. J. A. Monro, R. Leon, and B. K. Puri, "The Risk of Contamination in Bone Broth Diets," *Medical Hypotheses* 80, no. 4 (April 2013): 389–390, doi:10.1016/j.mehy.2012.12.026, accessed January 30, 2018.

21. K. Daniel, "Chicken Soup with Lead? Looking into a Controversy," Dr. Kaayla Daniel: The Naughty Nutritionist, 2013, http://drkaayladaniel.com/boning-up-is-broth -contaminated-with-lead/, accessed January 30, 2018.

22. "The BEST Article on Glyphosate with Comments from Jeffrey Smith," Institute for Responsible Technology, February 9, 2017, http://responsibletechnology.org/best-article -glyphosate-comments-jeffrey-smith/, accessed June 26, 2017.

23. J. L. Phillips, W. D. Winters, and L. Rutledge, "In Vitro Exposure to Electromagnetic Fields: Changes in Tumour Cell Properties," *International Journal of Radiation Biology and Related Studies in Physics, Chemistry and Medicine* 49, no. 3 (1985): 463–469, doi:10.1080/09553008514552681, accessed October 24, 2017.

24. "Quotes from Experts," Electromagnetichealth.org, July 18, 2010, http://electro magnetichealth.org/quotes-from-experts/, accessed June 26, 2017.

25. V. Burke, "Shungite: The Electropollution Solution," January 9, 2018, www.shungite queen.com

26. *Powerwatch*, http://www.powerwatch.org.uk/, accessed June 26, 2017.

27. O. M. Amin, "Seasonal Prevalence of Intestinal Parasites in the United States During 2000," *American Journal of Tropical Medicine and Hygiene* 66, no. 6 (2002): 799–803, doi:10.4269/ajtmh.2002.66.799, accessed June 26, 2017.

28. L. M. Stinton and E. A. Shaffer, "Epidemiology of Gallbladder Disease: Cholelithiasis and Cancer," *Gut and Liver* 6, no. 2 (2012): 172–187, doi:10.5009/gnl.2012.6.2.172, accessed June 26, 2017.

29. "What Is Biotoxin Illness?" Biotoxin Journey, December 3, 2014, http://biotoxinjourney.com/what-is-biotoxin-illness/, accessed June 26, 2017.

30. A. L. Gittleman, "Medical Mysteries Solved with 6 Strands of Hair?" annlouise.com, February 20, 2015.

31. Environmental Working Group, http://www.ewg.org/, accessed June 26, 2017.

32. W. Chowanadisai et al., "Pyrroloquinoline Quinone Stimulates Mitochondrial Biogenesis Through cAMP Response Element-Binding Protein Phosphorylation and Increased PGC-1α Expression," *Journal of Biological Chemistry* 285, no. 1 (2010): 142–152, doi:10.1074/jbc.M109.030130, accessed January 18, 2018.

CHAPTER 7: DETOX YOUR KITCHEN

1. Sadettin Turhan, "Aluminium Contents in Baked Meats Wrapped in Aluminium Foil," *Meat Science* 74, no. 4 (2006): 644–647, doi:10.1016/j.meatsci.2006.03.031, accessed June 23, 2017.

2. C. A. Full, and F. M. Parkins, "Effect of Cooking Vessel Composition on Fluoride," *Journal of Dental Research* 54, no. 1 (1975): 192, doi:10.1177/00220345750540012501, accessed June 23, 2017.

3. Truman Lewis, "Study Finds Teflon Chemical in Newborns' Umbilical Cords," Consumer Affairs, February 21, 2017, https://www.consumeraffairs.com/news04/2006/02/teflon_umbilical.html, accessed June 23, 2017.

4. Chun Z. Yang, "Estrogen Activity in Plastic Products: Yang et al. Respond," *Environmental Health Perspectives* 119, no. 9 (2011), doi:10.1289/ehp.1103894r, accessed June 23, 2017.

5. "Electromagnetic Fields (EMF) & Public Health: Microwave Ovens," World Health Organization, February 2005, http://www.who.int/peh-emf/publications/facts/info_microwaves/en/, accessed June 23, 2017.

6. D. F. George, M. M. Bilek, and D. R. Mckenzie,"Non-Thermal Effects in the Microwave Induced Unfolding of Proteins Observed by Chaperone Binding," *Bioelectromagnetics* 29, no. 4 (2008): 324–330, doi:10.1002/bem.20382, accessed June 23, 2017.

7. "DNA and the Microwave Effect," RF Safe, Penn State University, January 20, 2001, https://www.rfsafe.com/dna-and-the-microwave-effect/, accessed June 23, 2017.

8. F. Vallejo, F. A. Tomás-Barberán, and C. García-Viguera, "Phenolic Compound Contents in Edible Parts of Broccoli Inflorescences After Domestic Cooking," *Journal of the Science of Food and Agriculture* 83, no. 14 (2003): 1511–1516, doi:10.1002/jsfa.1585, accessed June 23, 2017.

9. R. Quan et al., "Effects of Microwave Radiation on Anti-Infective Factors in Human Milk," *Pediatrics* 89, no. 4, part 1 (1992): 667–669, https://www.ncbi.nlm.nih.gov/pubmed/1557249, accessed June 23, 2017.

10. "Microwave Oven and Microwave Cooking Overview," Powerwatch, http://www.powerwatch.org.uk/rf/microwaves.asp, accessed June 23, 2017.

CHAPTER 8: THE 4-DAY RADICAL INTENSIVE CLEANSE

1. C. Sandoval-Acuña, J. Ferreira, and H. Speisky, "Polyphenols and Mitochondria: An Update on Their Increasingly Emerging ROS-Scavenging Independent Actions," *Archives of Biochemistry and Biophysics* 559 (2014): 75–90, doi:10.1016/j.abb.2014.05.017, accessed November 1, 2017.

2. "Lose Your Worst," *First for Women Magazine*, June 19, 2017, 28–31.

3. C. A. Thaiss, "Persistent Microbiome Alterations Modulate the Rate of Post-Dieting Weight Regain," *Nature* 540, no. 7634 (2016): 544–551, doi:10.1038/nature20796, accessed June 22, 2017.

4. M. C. Fogarty et al., "Acute and Chronic Watercress Supplementation Attenuates Exercise-Induced Peripheral Mononuclear Cell DNA Damage and Lipid Peroxidation," *British Journal of Nutrition* 109, no. 2 (2012): 293–301, doi:10.1017/s0007114512000992, accessed January 29, 2018.

5. "Watercress," LifeExtension.com, http://www.lifeextension.com/magazine/2007/11/sf_watercress/Page-01, accessed November 1, 2017.

CHAPTER 9: THE 21-DAY RADICAL REBOOT—AND BEYOND

1. N. Hongu and D. S. Sachan, "Caffeine, Carnitine and Choline Supplementation of Rats Decreases Body Fat and Serum Leptin Concentration as Does Exercise," *Journal of Nutrition* 130, no. 2 (January 2000): 152–157, accessed January 16, 2018.

2. W. J. Pasman et al., "The Effect of Korean Pine Nut Oil on In Vitro CCK Release, on Appetite Sensations and on Gut Hormones in Post-Menopausal Overweight Women," *Lipids in Health and Disease* 7, no. 10 (March 2008), doi:10.1186/1476-511x-7-10, accessed July 10, 2017.

3. S. Park et al., "Korean Pine Nut Oil Attenuated Hepatic Triacylglycerol Accumulation in High-Fat Diet-Induced Obese Mice," *Nutrients* 8, no. 1 (2016), doi:10.3390/nu8010059, accessed July 10, 2017.

4. "Dandy Tummy Bitters Recipe," Mountain Rose Herbs Blog, https://blog.mountainroseherbs.com/dandy-tummy-bitters-recipe, accessed June 22, 2017.

5. B. Rubik, "How Does Pork Prepared in Various Ways Affect the Blood," Weston A. Price Foundation, October 12, 2011, https://www.westonaprice.org/health-topics/food-features/how-does-pork-prepared-in-various-ways-affect-the-blood/, accessed November 3, 2017.

6. "The Down Side to High Oxalates—Problems with Sulfate, B6, Gut, and Methylation," *Beyond MTHFR*, March 21, 2016, http://www.beyondmthfr.com/side-high-oxalates-problems-sulfate-b6-gut-methylation/, accessed June 22, 2017.

7. Katz, *Wild Fermentation*; Sally Fallon et al., *Nourishing Traditions: The Cookbook That Challenges Politically Correct Nutrition and the Diet Dictocrats* (Washington, DC: NewTrends Publishing, Inc., 2005).

8. Valerie Burke, "Val's Naturally Fermented Veggies," *Panther Speak*, February 2015, *https://pantherspeak.wordpress.com/*; Valerie Burke, "Val's Naturally Fermented Pickles," *Panther Speak*, August 2015, https://pantherspeak.wordpress.com.

9. Su-Chen Ho, Tsai Tzung-Hsun, Tsai Po-Jung, and Lin Chih-Cheng, "Protective Capacities of Certain Spices Against Peroxynitrite-Mediated Biomolecular Damage," *Food and Chemical Toxicology* 46, no. 3 (2008): 920–928, doi:10.1016/j.fct.2007.10.028, accessed June 22, 2017.

10. "Cancer-Fighting Properties of Horseradish Revealed," *ScienceDaily*, May 17, 2016, https://www.sciencedaily.com/releases/2016/05/160517122054.htm, accessed June 22, 2017.

11. Kento Kitada et al., "High Salt Intake Reprioritizes Osmolyte and Energy Metabolism for Body Fluid Conservation," *Journal of Clinical Investigation* (May 18, 2017), https://www.jci.org/articles/view/88532, accessed June 22, 2017.

12. Robert H. Lustig, et al., "Isocaloric Fructose Restriction and Metabolic Improvement in Children with Obesity and Metabolic Syndrome," *Obesity* 24, no. 2 (2015): 453–460, doi:10.1002/oby.21371, accessed June 22, 2017.

13. "Glycemic Index for Sweeteners," http://www.sugar-and-sweetener-guide.com /glycemic-index-for-sweeteners.html, accessed June 22, 2017.

14. Susana Genta et al., "Yacon Syrup: Beneficial Effects on Obesity and Insulin Resistance in Humans," *Clinical Nutrition* 28, no. 2 (2009): 182–187, doi:10.1016/j.clnu.2009.01.013, accessed June 22, 2017.

15. Aleksandra M. Mirończuk et al., "A Two-Stage Fermentation Process of Erythritol Production by Yeast Y. Lipolytica from Molasses and Glycerol," *Bioresource Technology* 198 (2015): 445–455, doi:10.1016/j.biortech.2015.09.008, accessed June 22, 2017.

16. "The Healthiest Coffee in the World," Dr. Sircus, April 10, 2017, http://drsircus.com /seed-nutrition/the-healthiest-coffee-in-the-world/, accessed June 22, 2017.

17. P. Shokouh et al., "A Combination of Coffee Compounds Shows Insulin-Sensitizing and Hepatoprotective Effects in a Rat Model of Diet-Induced Metabolic Syndrome," *Nutrients* 10, no. 1 (December 2017): pii E6; doi: 10.3390/nu10010006, accessed January 16, 2018.

18. I. Park et al., "Effects of Subacute Ingestion of Chlorogenic Acids on Sleep Architecture and Energy Metabolism Through Activity of the Autonomic Nervous System: A Randomised, Placebo-Controlled, Double-Blinded Cross-Over Trial," *British Journal of Nutrition* 117, no. 7 (April 2017): 979–984, doi: 10.1017/S0007114517000587, accessed January 16, 2018.

19. Haruna Baba et al., "Studies of Anti-Inflammatory Effects of Rooibos Tea in Rats," *Pediatrics International* 51, no. 5 (2009): 700–704, doi:10.1111/j.1442-200x.2009.02835.x, accessed June 22, 2017; South African Rooibos Council, Rooibos Council, http://sarooibos .co.za/, accessed June 7, 2017.

20. J. Gill, "The Effects of Moderate Alcohol Consumption on Female Hormone Levels and Reproductive Function," *Alcohol and Alcoholism* 35, no. 5 (2000): 417–423, doi:10.1093/ alcalc/35.5.417, accessed June 22, 2017; J. S. Gavaler, "Alcoholic Beverages as a Source of Estrogens," *Alcohol Health and Research World* 22, no. 3 (1998): 220–227, PMID:15706799, https://pubs.niaaa.nih.gov/publications/arh22-3/220.pdf, accessed June 20, 2017.

21. "Cool Temperature Alters Human Fat and Metabolism," National Institutes of Health, May 15, 2015, https://www.nih.gov/news-events/nih-research-matters/cool -temperature-alters-human-fat-metabolism, accessed June 26, 2017.

INDEX

yellow
kite

books to help you live a good life

Join the conversation and tell
us how you live a #goodlife

🐦 @yellowkitebooks
📘 YellowKiteBooks
📌 Yellow Kite Books
📷 YellowKiteBooks